# CARE and
# COVENANT

# CARE and COVENANT

## A Jewish Bioethic of Responsibility

*Jason Weiner*

Georgetown University Press / Washington, DC

The publisher is not responsible for third-party websites or their content. URL links were active at time of publication.

Library of Congress Cataloging-in-Publication Data

Names: Weiner, Jason, author.
Title: Care and covenant : a Jewish bioethic of responsibility / Jason Weiner.
Description: Washington, DC : Georgetown University Press, 2022. | Includes bibliographical references and index.
Identifiers: LCCN 2022013310 (print) | LCCN 2022013311 (ebook) | ISBN 9781647123178 (hardcover) | ISBN 9781647123185 (paperback) | ISBN 9781647123192 (ebook)
Subjects: LCSH: Medical ethics—Religious aspects—Judaism. | Bioethics—Religious aspects—Judaism.
Classification: LCC R727.57 .W46 2022 (print) | LCC R727.57 (ebook) | DDC 174.2—dc23/eng/20220616
LC record available at https://lccn.loc.gov/2022013310
LC ebook record available at https://lccn.loc.gov/2022013311

∞ This paper meets the requirements of ANSI/NISO Z39.48-1992 (Permanence of Paper).

24 23          9 8 7 6 5 4 3

Printed in the United States of America

Cover image by Terry Schoonhoven. The image is taken from a mural titled *Jewish Contributions to Medicine* which Schoonhoven completed in 1999 for the Harvey Morse Auditorium at Cedars-Sinai Medical Center in Los Angeles. The man seated at the table is Dr. Jesse Lazear, the focus of this book's first chapter.
Interior design by Paul Hotvedt.
Production Assistant, Jenna Galberg.

*To my family and all those who give of themselves to make the world a little bit better.*

# Contents

# Preface

This book is intended for health care practitioners, bioethicists, and public health officials of all religions and backgrounds who are searching for meaningful values to help inform their practices and policymaking. It will likely also be very relevant to the work of chaplains and clergy. In recent years many theologians have become less interested in contributing to public discourse, and many secular bioethicists have become less open to input from religious perspectives, which has been detrimental to each discipline.[1] Theologians, and the Jewish tradition, have important perspectives that can contribute significantly to crucial contemporary health care deliberations. This is not to suggest that people who are not Jewish should feel any sense of obligation to follow the Jewish ethical tradition but simply that it may provide useful insights and guidance that can inform one's moral decision-making and perspectives. Religious traditions have a rich history of providing comprehensive, wise insight to societal dilemmas and have the potential to significantly expand and benefit the field of bioethics. With this goal in mind, this book is an attempt to show how numerous classic Jewish texts, history, and ideas have meaningful things to say about some of the most urgent societal debates in the world of medicine today.[2] Rabbis, scholars, and those interested in how Judaism can be effectively applied to real-world deliberations will thus also find this work valuable.

This book not only is about applying classical Jewish values to bioethical dilemmas but also seeks specifically to develop an approach that is primarily informed by personal and communal obligations and social responsibilities. Indeed, some contemporary thinkers argue that because Jewish values focus on requirements, obligations, and commandments, Judaism's approach can be understood as an "ethics of responsibility."[3] This approach is found in Jewish perspectives on modern bioethical dilemmas as well.[4] Dr. Benjamin Freedman, a clinical bioethicist and scholar, developed what he called an "ethics of duty" based on this perspective, in which he argued that the Western approach to bioethics focuses on patients' *rights* and their autonomy, but a Jewish approach must be based more on one's *obligations* toward patients.[5] Freedman's work was traditional in that it aligns with classical rulings of Jewish law, but it also led him to unique and original conclusions, many of which I find highly compelling.

Unfortunately, just as Freedman was fully articulating this duty-based approach to Jewish bioethics, he died at the young age of forty-six, and he was never able to fully develop these ideas.[6] More recently, the former chief rabbi of the United Kingdom, Rabbi Lord Jonathan Sacks, an internationally renowned theologian and moral thinker, articulated a philosophical approach that closely resembled Freedman's. For many years I found Rabbi Sacks's writings to be beautiful articulations of a call to action that profoundly resonated with my work in the hospital and that inspired me deeply. Although Rabbi Sacks didn't focus specifically on medical ethics, it seems to me that many of his core insights (many of which are described below) could be effectively applied to numerous areas of medical ethics—sometimes with deep potential for addressing several challenging dilemmas. As I was writing this book, in the fall of 2020, I prepared a list of philosophical and practical questions related to the various issues addressed in this book that I planned to discuss with Rabbi Sacks. Unfortunately, just as I was attempting to reach out to him, he also suddenly died an untimely death.

Although I do not come near these giants of ethics and scholarship, this book represents my own attempt to advance conversations on these important issues by applying classic Jewish values and requirements as well as examples from Jewish history to some of the most challenging contemporary bioethical dilemmas regularly faced by patients, hospitals, and society at large. In undertaking this task, in the spirit of Dr. Freedman, Rabbi Sacks, and others, I hope to further develop a Jewish bioethic of responsibility, advancing new, relevant approaches that can encourage health care providers to remain dedicated to preventing harm and providing compassionate care to all based on these inspiring and timeless values. Neither of these great thinkers are quoted in every chapter of this book, but their approaches have inspired my thinking throughout.

The perspective that I personally bring to this discussion is that of a practitioner who has been working in a hospital with patients and medical staff for almost fifteen years, observing and taking part in the intricacies of the various dilemmas that arise, how decisions are made, and what factors can go into making improvements. As a board-certified chaplain, my perspective focuses primarily on compassionate, nonjudgmental care for the whole person, mind, body, and soul. This approach is slightly different from that of some of these "responsibility ethicists" by further emphasizing the central role of compassion. Further, since I have earned a doctorate in clinical bioethics, I am also informed by the analytical, philosophical, and evidence-based scholarship that has helped to frame many of these and similar discussions. Last, I am an Orthodox rabbi. While I focus primarily on Jewish sources that were written before any denominations existed and I strive to write in a way that is broad-minded and inclusive of all Jews—indeed, all humanity—it is important to point out that the traditional codes of Jewish law and responsa literature are what most inform my thinking on these matters.

Bridging these various disciplines and perspectives is not simple. Jewish bioethics often focuses on rulings of Jewish law based on interpretation and application of specific authoritative texts, classical sources, and precedents. Bioethicists, on the other hand, tend to derive their discourse from philosophical analysis and application of "first principles." And chaplains focus on respecting the unique narrative of each individual and providing care from within that individual's own unique perspective. This book attempts to synthesize these approaches by showing how rulings of Jewish law interact with principles of bioethics and by teasing out the various rabbinical rulings to develop the Jewish bioethical values that underlie each ruling. I then suggest ways in which these values might be effectively applied in the clinical setting.

My previous books provide brief summaries of issues and practical guidance. By contrast, this book more fully examines core ideas and underlying theories. Furthermore, my earlier works summarize the rulings of Jewish legal authorities, without presenting my own opinions. By contrast, although I rely on thinkers much greater than myself in this book, I also suggest my own original ideas based on this compassionate, duty-based paradigm. This book is not intended to serve as an exhaustive survey of all of Jewish bioethics. The topics explored in this book are primarily those that I have found to be very common and challenging in my clinical practice and to which insufficient attention has been paid in recent Jewish writings as well as those that I have something practical to add to the dialogue.

The issues are complex, and the principles aren't always easy to apply to every scenario. Each chapter of this book explores such questions as the following: Are we expected to risk our lives on behalf of others? When we can help only a limited number of people, how do we prioritize? What are the obligations and expectations of a society or government? Are issues of cultural sensitivity relevant in how we discharge our obligations to others? What should we do when obligations for others violate our own moral principles or commitments? Are there limits to how far one can be expected to go for others? These and other issues are addressed in this book as I attempt to describe a meaningful Jewish bioethic of responsibility for our times.

## NOTES

1. Michael McCarthy, Mary Homan, and Michael Rozier, "There's No Harm in Talking: Re-establishing the Relationship between Theological and Secular Bioethics," *American Journal of Bioethics* 20, no. 12 (2020): 12.

2. On the importance of sharing the messages of Jewish values with all humanity, see Jonathan Sacks, *Future Tense: Jews, Judaism, and Israel in the Twenty-First Century* (New York: Schocken, 2009), 6–10, 129–30. Sacks once lamented that Jewish medical ethics is primarily only about private decisions between patient and doctor. Jonathan Sacks, "Torah Umadda: The Unwritten Chapter," *Tradition* 53, no. 3 (Summer 2021): 201. This book, however, seeks to demonstrate how Jewish medical ethics can indeed address concerns of the public domain as well.

3. Walter S. Wurzburger, *Ethics of Responsibility: Pluralistic Approaches to Covenantal Ethics* (Philadelphia: Jewish Publication Society, 1994), 15; Jonathan Sacks, *To Heal a Fractured World: The Ethics of Responsibility* (New York: Schocken, 2005), 183. See also Erich Fromm, *You Shall Be as Gods: A Radical Interpretation of the Old Testament and Its Tradition* (New York: Holt, Rinehart and Winston, 1966), 56; and Harry Redner, *Ethical Life: The Past Present of Ethical Cultures* (Lanham, MD: Rowman & Littlefield, 2001).

4. Immanuel Jakobovits, *The Timely and the Timeless: Jews, Judaism and Society in a Storm-Tossed Decade* (London: Vallentine, Mitchell, 1977), 128; Fred Rosner, "Managed Care: The Jewish View," in *Biomedical Ethics and Jewish Law* (Hoboken, NJ: Ktav, 2001), 518; and A. Steinberg, *HaRefuah KeHalakhah*, vol. 1 (Jerusalem: printed by the author, 2017), 159.

5. Benjamin Freedman, *Duty and Healing: Foundations of a Jewish Bioethic* (New York: Routledge, 1999), 12, 35, 48–54. In fact, Dr. Freedman goes so far as to argue that in some cases Judaism does not see a conflict between rights and duties but rather there are only duties: the duty of a physician to care for the patient, and the duty of the patient to care for their own body (302). Bioethicist Laurie Zoloth, PhD, articulates a very compelling Jewish bioethic of responsibility based on the work of Dr. Freedman, as well as Emmanuel Levinas and numerous biblical and rabbinic texts, particularly in chapters 7 and 9 of her book *Second Texts/Second Opinions: Essays toward a Jewish Bioethics* (Oxford: Oxford University Press, 2022).

6. François Baylis and Charles Weijer, "Remembering Benjamin Freedman (1951–1997)," *Hastings Center Report* 27, no. 3 (May/June 1997): 48.

# Acknowledgments

Much of the work for this book was done as part of my doctorate in Clinical Bioethics at Loyola University, Chicago, and I owe a tremendous debt of gratitude to all of my incredible professors there, particularly my doctoral advisers, Nanette Elster, JD, MPH; Kayhan Parsi, JD, PhD, HEC-C; and Katherine Wasson, PhD, MPH, HEC-C. I have significantly revised, expanded, and updated the material since preparing it for my doctorate, and I am especially grateful to the expert proofreading and feedback of Stuart Finder, PhD; Paula Van Gelder, BCC; Nechama Unterman; and the incredible team at Georgetown University Press, who carefully and insightfully commented on every single page of this book.

I also appreciate all my unparalleled colleagues in the Spiritual Care department at Cedars-Sinai and the exceptional support and guidance of my wonderful supervisor, Jonathan Schreiber, MSBA, MBA, MAEd. It is also truly an honor and privilege to be the rabbi of a dynamic and passionate synagogue, Knesset Israel of Beverlywood, whose intelligent and thoughtful members constantly inspire me to grow and continually thirst for deeper insights and gave me important feedback as I presented each of these chapters as lectures.

I would also like to acknowledge the publications that allowed me to republish revised and expanded editions of my articles that appeared in their publications: *Esther in America* (Maggid Books), *Jewish End-of-Life Care in a Virtual Age* (Albion-Andalus Books), canopyforum.org, *Hakira*, *AMA Journal of Ethics*, *Rambam Maimonides Medical Journal*, *Journal of Religion and Health*, and *Journal of Jewish Ethics*.

I would also like to thank God for enabling me to have the health, time, and ability to do the work necessary to complete this book. Finally, and most importantly, I would like to thank my wife, Lauren, for being my life partner and inspiration and for giving me the time and encouragement to complete the book while raising a family and working multiple jobs.

This book would not be what it is without all of the incredible support and assistance of those mentioned above, although of course, any mistakes remain mine alone.

# Introduction

The focus on obligations and responsibilities goes back to the very origins of Judaism. While it goes without saying that there are many very good people in the world of all religions and of no religion, one of the most influential sources of inspiration for helping others is the Bible. "The Bible is God's call to human responsibility," argues Rabbi Jonathan Sacks.[1] He claims that the Hebrew Bible (in particular) is not the cry of humanity to God but God's cry to each of us, with human responsibility being its single greatest overarching theme.[2] In fact, Rabbi Sacks further suggests that the Torah introduces a number of different types of responsibility in its opening chapters. It begins with the story of Adam and Eve, in which humanity is granted the freedom to choose, yet every character in the story blames the other, teaching the lesson and value of "personal responsibility."

When Adam and Eve sinned, God called out, "Where are you?" This call was not directed only to them; it echoes in every generation.[3] Their son Cain is punished for killing his brother, Abel, and claims that he need not be concerned with the welfare of anyone but himself, a denial that is rejected, hence introducing the notion of "moral responsibility," of having responsibility not for oneself alone but for others as well. Noah then fails to express any concern for the society around him, hinting at the value of social responsibility.[4] Next comes the story of the Tower of Babel, with the theme that all are accountable to something or someone beyond themselves, which relates to the very nature of human existence or "ontological responsibility." Then Abraham is assigned the task of transmitting ideas of monotheism and morality to a people, highlighting the centrality of "national responsibility."[5] There is also a type of responsibility that goes beyond only members of one's own faith or community. Abraham goes on to demonstrate human solidarity by rushing to care for his noon-time visitors (Gen. 18:1–8) and advocating for the people of Sodom (18:23–32). Once Abraham had the courage to challenge God, his descendants learned to challenge injustice from human rulers as well.[6] Hence we see Moses coming to the defense of seven Midianite daughters, expressing outrage at no one coming to the rescue when an Egyptian overseer beats a Hebrew slave, and attempting to make peace when two Hebrew slaves quarrel with each other (Ex. 2:11–20). These actions represent "collective responsibility."[7]

By the time we get to the book of Deuteronomy, we are introduced to a unique vision of society that creates structures of cooperation through a pledge or bond of mutual fidelity, individual and collective responsibility, merging all citizens into a freely chosen set of obligations. This biblical form of acceptance of responsibility by each member of society became known as a covenant, which is the basis of the common good and an ethic of responsibility.[8]

The stories of the Bible demonstrate a process of gradually transferring the initiative from God to humanity. The narratives reveal a process of humanity's oscillating between dependence and rebelliousness, until humanity gradually learns to honor God by accepting responsibility.[9] This progression culminates toward the very end of the Hebrew Bible, in the book of Esther, with the empowering and dramatic ultimatum that Mordechai poses to Esther: "If you are silent at this time, relief and deliverance will come from elsewhere . . . but who knows whether it was not all for this moment that you have attained royalty?" (Esther 4:14).

It is this question, argues Rabbi Sacks, that God's cry constantly poses to all of us: "Yes, if we do not do it, someone else may. But we will then have failed to understand why we are here and what we are summoned to do."[10]

This value is not only demonstrated by biblical stories but also by many biblical laws and values that demand communal and personal responsibility for the common good.[11] This approach is also hinted at in the Aleinu prayer, which is recited at the conclusion of all Jewish prayer services, three times a day, which suggests that it is our duty "letakein olam bemalkhut Sha-dai," to "perfect the world under the sovereignty of God." The classic eighteenth-century work of character development, the *Mesillat Yesharim* ("The Path of the Just"), opens with a chapter titled "A Person's Obligation in the World," making the striking point that "the foundation of true piety and the root of perfect service of God is formed by a person clarifying to themselves what their obligation is in the world and toward what goal one should direct their outlook and ambition in everything that they strive for during their lifetime."[12]

A profound insight of my great rabbi and teacher, Rabbi Asher Weiss, a leading authority in Jewish law and the rabbinic decisor of Shaare Zedek Medical Center in Jerusalem, sharply demonstrates the extent of these expectations. The Torah commands judges "not to fear anyone" (Deut. 1:17). The rabbis explained that this includes a situation in which a judge may fear that one of the litigants might even try to kill the judge. The judge is nevertheless required by Jewish law to render judgment in the case. However, given that Jewish law rules that protecting life sets aside most of the Torah, how could there be such an expectation of the judge? Rabbi Weiss explains that this is because there are certain essential professionals who serve the community, such as judges, health care professionals, and firefighters, whom the Torah requires to expose themselves to significant danger if necessary for the sake of the public welfare.[13] We thus see that the Hebrew Bible, beginning with God's rhetorical call to all of humanity, "Where are you?" and continuing with the development of Jewish law throughout the ages, is a sustained challenge to recognize responsibilities and take the appropriate actions. The world will not get better on its own.

## APPLICATION TO ETHICAL THEORY

Although contemporary society often emphasizes individual *rights*, and traditional Jewish values focus on *obligations*, this does not mean that there is no place for rights in Judaism.[14] God's intervention to deliver the people of Israel out of Egyptian slavery is seen as a quintessential act of defense of human rights, which is rooted in all of humanity having been created in the image of God.[15] Furthermore, one of the crucial lessons of the Holocaust is that medical education and medical ethics without focus on respect for individual human rights can lead to the most heinous abuses of medical expertise.[16] Rights and obligations are closely connected. For example, according to traditional Jewish law, there is a right to keep and protect one's property from theft, just as there is a correlative obligation not to steal from others. Similarly, there is an obligation to rescue persons in danger, just as there is a correlative right to be rescued from danger.[17] Every right has a corresponding duty, just as many duties have corresponding rights.[18] The important question is which is primary. While there are "rights-based" moral theories that argue that human rights come first, Jewish perspectives usually maintain that obligations are more fundamental.[19] Rights are the result of these responsibilities, which create the moral commitments to ensure that individual rights exist and are honored.[20] So while Judaism certainly affirms that all people possess some nonnegotiable human dignity and rights, our duties exceed our rights, so our primary focus must be on our responsibility to create and sustain a society which honors that dignity of each person.[21]

This focus on obligations also emphasizes expectations of altruistic love for others, giving over receiving, and being concerned with other people's needs rather than one's own entitlements.[22] That is why the Hebrew word for responsibility is *achrayut* which comes from *acher*, meaning "other."[23] Jewish ethics requires us to be sensitive to the needs of others and help enable them to experience dignity. Taking responsibility is not only an internal value; it is also a response to an obligation to care for someone outside of us, focusing on communal needs, with others' rights following our obligations. Jewish values thus recognize both rights and obligations, but the primary focus is on obligations.[24]

## INSPIRATION FOR RESPONSIBILITY

When I was in college, I was told an unforgettable story that has become one of the most inspiring stories that I have ever heard. It summarizes the essence of what I believe an ethic of responsibility is all about.[25] It is a simple and perhaps even somewhat common personal account, but it resonated with me in a profound way and may have changed the trajectory of my life. It is a story of a young high school student who had a dream. She wanted to help others and make a difference in the world, and she became very focused. She took advanced classes and got involved in extracurricular activities. Early on she struggled, and even failed a few classes, but she worked with tutors to help her get the best grades that she could. Sometimes she would stay home to study when her friends made plans or there was a school event, because she had a dream. She aced her SATs and got into her preferred college, where she stepped up her level of dedication.

She often consulted her professors during their office hours to make sure she fully understood the material, stayed up late studying, and didn't let anything deter her from her goal. As her years in college passed, she jumped at the opportunity to take on enriching internships while working even harder in her classes, as she sensed her dream coming closer to fruition. Although different life distractions came up, she managed to remain focused and enthusiastic about her studies, because she had a dream. Before she knew it, she was accepted into one of the best medical schools in the world.

On the first day of medical school classes, one of her professors told the students to "look around, because most of you won't keep up with our rigorous standards, and only the most devoted will graduate!" She did not let that negative pronouncement deter her. Some of her classes were especially difficult, and at first she didn't get the best grades. She routinely stayed up well into the night studying, sometimes all night. She joined study groups and attended seminars to enhance her learning. She was frequently exhausted, but she excelled because she had a dream. She graduated at the top of her class and was assigned her first residency. The dream was becoming a reality, and she could hardly wait.

Her first rotation was in the emergency room. She was literally shaking with excitement as she struggled to put on her scrubs and white coat. As she walked through the staff entrance of the emergency room, with tears of joy and anticipation in her eyes, she encountered a friend from medical school. He looked horrible, as if he were in some sort of daze. He blurted out, "You don't want to go in there, it's horrible! People are so sick, there is blood everywhere, terrible injuries, children suffering, people are dying, it's . . . it's . . . it's a nightmare!"

With empathy, but in shock, she looked at her friend and responded, "Do you mean to tell me that people are in grave need of our help, and you are calling *that* a nightmare? We are trained to help them. We can help them. That is not a nightmare. This . . . this . . . this is my dream!" It was all for this moment. And she confidently, but humbly, walked into the emergency room and began saving lives.

We all have the opportunity to give and impact the world in different ways. The first step is acknowledging our responsibility to do so, followed by determining the best method for each of us. It is my hope and prayer that the discussions in this book will help you clarify your own personal approach to these crucial matters.

## NOTES

1. Jonathan Sacks, *To Heal a Fractured World: The Ethics of Responsibility* (New York: Schocken, 2005), 134.

2. Sacks. Elsewhere he phrases this as "Judaism is God's call to responsibility." Jonathan Sacks, *Lessons in Leadership: A Weekly Reading of the Jewish Bible* (New Milford, CT: Maggid, 2015), 95.

3. Immanuel Etkes, *Rabbi Shneur Zalman of Liady: The Origins of Chabad Hasidism* (Waltham, MA: Brandeis University Press, 2015), 181. Biblical translations based on Rabbi Sacks's.

4. In *To Heal a Fractured World*, Rabbi Sacks refers to the responsibility taught by Noah as "collective responsibility," but I have chosen to refer to it here as "social responsibility" because in a later work, quoted below, he refers to "collective responsibility" in a slightly different context. This was a question I had intended to ask Rabbi Sacks about.

5. Sacks, *To Heal a Fractured World*, 144–45.

6. Sacks, 144–45.

7. Sacks, *Lessons in Leadership*, 22.

8. Jonathan Sacks, *Covenant & Conversation, a Weekly Reading of the Jewish Bible: Deuteronomy; Renewal of the Sinai Covenant* (New Milford, CT: Maggid, 2019), 5–6, 16, 59; and Jonathan Sacks, *Ceremony & Celebration: Introduction to the Holidays* (New Milford, CT: Maggid, 2017), 295. For this reason, Rabbi Sacks argues that "the basis of social order in Judaism is not power but collective responsibility" (294).

9. Sacks, *To Heal a Fractured World*, 155.

10. Sacks, 28. Rabbi Sacks beautifully summarizes this elsewhere by stating "It is not what God does for us but what we do for God that allows us to reach dignity and responsibility." Sacks, *Lessons in Leadership*, 97.

11. Such as "Do not stand idly by" (Lev. 19, *Shulchan Arukh*, CM 425); "Love your neighbor as yourself" (Lev. 19, Rambam, *Hilkhot Avel* 14:1); and "You must open your hand and lend to the poor" (Deut. 15:8, *Shulchan Arukh*, YD 247–52). Furthermore, Rabbi Sacks argues that some aspects of collective responsibility were simply taken for granted during the biblical period, when all citizens were connected and lived in proximity of each other. After the destruction of the Temple, however, as the Jews went into exile, the rabbis had to codify this sense of shared bond and responsibility by teaching that "all Israel are responsible for each other." Jonathan Sacks, *Future Tense: Jews, Judaism, and Israel in the Twenty-First Century* (New York: Schocken, 2009), 40–45.

12. Rabbi M. C. Luzzatto, *Mesillat Yesharim: The Path of the Upright* (New York: Feldheim Publishers, 1993), ch. 1.

13. Responsa *Minchat Asher* 3:121(2); *Minchat Asher–Magefat HaKorona* (Jerusalem: printed by the author, 2021), 8(2).

14. *Mikhtav MeEliyahu*, 1:77n. See also Robert M. Cover, "Obligation: A Jewish Jurisprudence of the Social Order," *Journal of Law and Religion* 5, no. 1 (1987): 65–74; Martha Minow, Michael Ryan, and Austin Sarat, eds., *Narrative, Violence, and the Law: The Essays of Robert Cover* (Ann Arbor: University of Michigan Press, 1995), 239–40; and Immanuel Jakobovits, *The Timely and the Timeless: Jews, Judaism and Society in a Storm-Tossed Decade* (London: Vallentine, Mitchell, 1977), 128, who demonstrate that the ultimate expression of Judaism is in its incumbent obligations, not in individual rights, and that it is an obligation-centered legal system, which is why Judaism has so many biblical Hebrew terms for "obligations" and "duties" but no word for "rights." Although some Jewish thinkers disagree with this statement (see note 20 below), Rabbi J. Sacks argues that the Bible has no word for "rights" because its moral vision is set forth entirely in terms of duties, obligation, responsibilities, and commands, but rights are presupposed. For example, the command to pursue justice entails the right to a fair trial and the rule of law. The duty to set aside portions of the harvest for the poor represents a right to their welfare. Jonathan Sacks, *The Home We Build Together: Moving beyond Multiculturalism* (London: Continuum, 2007), 132. See also Jonathan Sacks, *Covenant & Conversation, a Weekly Reading of the Jewish Bible: Genesis* (New Milford, CT: Maggid, 2009), 75, 298–300; and a similar argument in Nahum Lamm, *Seventy Faces: Articles of Faith* (Hoboken, NJ: Ktav, 2002), 2:17.

15. Jonathan Sacks, *The Great Partnership: Science, Religion, and Search for Meaning* (New York: Schocken, 2011), 69. See elaboration of this point in Jonathan Sacks, *Covenant & Conversation, a Weekly Reading of the Jewish Bible: Exodus* (New Milford, CT: Maggid, 2010), 7. Rabbi Sacks also argues that the biblical story of the daughters of Tzlofhad and the claim for their inheritance is another example emphasizing the importance of communal and individual human rights in the Torah. Jonathan Sacks, *Covenant & Conversation, a Weekly Reading of the Jewish Bible: Numbers* (New Milford, CT: Maggid, 2017), 413–17. See also Jonathan Sacks, *Essays on Ethics: A Weekly Reading of the Jewish Bible* (New Milford, CT: Maggid, 2016), 190–91; and Sacks, *Future Tense*, 78. See also Itamar Rosensweig and Shua Mermelstein, "Rights and Duties in Jewish Law," *Touro Law Review* 37, no. 4 (2022): 2179–209. who argue at length that rights do play a central role in Jewish law, and that in some instances they are in fact primary.

16. Evelyne Shuster, "Fifty Years Later: The Significance of the Nuremberg Code," *New*

*England Journal of Medicine* 337 (1997): 1430; and Florian Bruns and Tessa Chelouche, "Lectures on Inhumanity: Teaching Medical Ethics in German Medical Schools under Nazism," *Annals of Internal Medicine* 166 (2017): 591–95. See also Shmuel P. Reis, Hedy S. Wald, and Paul Weindling, "The Holocaust, Medicine and Becoming a Physician: The Crucial Role of Education," *Israel Journal of Health Policy Research* 8, no. 55 (2019); Tessa Chelouche, "Teaching Hard Truths about Medicine and the Holocaust," *AMA Journal of Ethics* 23, no. 1 (2021): 59–63. This is true not only regarding medicine but also on a societal level since the Holocaust is also a terrifying reminder of the dangers of democracy/majority rule without protection of individual rights. David Novak, *Covenantal Rights: A Study in Jewish Political Theory* (Princeton, NJ: Princeton University Press, 2000), 204. Indeed, since 1945 the volume of human rights talk has risen to unprecedented levels as a reaction against the Nazi regime. Nigel Biggar, *What's Wrong with Rights?* (Oxford: Oxford University Press, 2020), 190.

17. See discussion in Tom L. Beauchamp and James F. Childress, *Principles of Biomedical Ethics*, 8th ed. (New York: Oxford University Press, 2019), 405. Rabbi Sacks argues that rights and obligations aren't always correlative, because they belong to two different systems: rights are legislated in law, whereas responsibilities are educated in the moral imagination/culture and can't always be legislated. Although a system of rights, Rabbi Sacks argues, must be accompanied by a culture of responsibility. Sacks, *Home We Build Together*, 132–33.

18. Some moral theologians are careful to emphasize that respect for human dignity suggests that any right implies a corresponding duty, but not all duties imply rights. For example, a legal right to freedom of speech implies a legal duty to tolerate someone saying things (within the law) that others don't like, but the speaker also has a moral duty not to abuse their legal right to free speech by deliberately insulting and provoking others. Thus, some duties do not imply rights, but all rights imply duties. Fundamental rights exist only when there is an agent capable of performing the corresponding duty, but duties can arise outside of rights. Therefore, it is duties that determine if, and how, rights can be exercised; see Biggar, *What's Wrong with Rights?*, 70, 93, 99–101, 329, 334.

19. Beauchamp and Childress, *Principles of Biomedical Ethics*, 407.

20. See, for example, extensive discussions in Sacks, *To Heal a Fractured World*, 183; Elliot N. Dorff, *To Do the Right and the Good: A Jewish Approach to Modern Social Ethics* (Philadelphia: Jewish Publication Society, 2002), 18–19; and Akiva Tatz, *World Mask* (Southfield, MI: Targum/Feldheim, 1995), 103–5. On the other hand, others argue that in Judaism, rights generate duties because it is God's rights that generate human duties, and, for example, the poor are in need before we have a duty to help them, which makes one's duty a response to their right to be helped. Novak, *Covenantal Rights*, 10, 25, 132. A similar argument, but without mention of "God's rights," is made in Haim Hermann Cohn, *Human Rights in Jewish Law* (New York: Ktav, 1984), 17fn. That said, these perspectives still recognize a difference between secular rights talk, which tends to focus on rights of the individual, and Judaism's focus on rights of the community. Novak, *Covenantal Rights*, 193–94.

21. Laurie Zoloth, *Second Texts/Second Opinions: Essays toward a Jewish Bioethics* (Oxford: Oxford University Press, 2022), ch. 5; and Sacks, *Essays on Ethics*, 211. Rabbi Sacks argues that this is also the position of Maimonides (*Guide to the Perplexed* 3:17) when he argues that cruelty to animals is not wrong because animals have rights but because we have duties, including

the duty not to be cruel, which promotes virtues in humans. Sacks, *Covenant & Conversation: Deuteronomy*, 199.

22. Philosopher Harry Redner refers to Jewish biblical ethics as "the ethic of love" in his *Ethical Life: The Past Present of Ethical Cultures* (Lanham, MD: Rowman & Littlefield, 2001), 50. See elaboration in Sacks, *Covenant & Conversation: Deuteronomy*, 95.

23. Sacks, *To Heal a Fractured World*, 144, 220.

24. Rabbi Sacks argues elsewhere that "rights" and "responsibilities" have not always been in opposition to one another. He demonstrates that "rights" used to refer to restrictions on government interventions, so that communities could exercise their moral *responsibilities* to each member of the community. Today, as communities and collective responsibility have weakened, the state has taken on more power. "Rights" talk in the West now refers to *personal entitlement* and demands on the state, such that communal responsibility and morality have been replaced by politics and impersonal government. Jonathan Sacks, *Morality: Restoring the Common Good in Divided Times* (New York: Basic, 2020), 119–25, 304–5; and Sacks, *Home We Build Together*, 60. Indeed, in many non-Western societies today, such as much of Asia and Africa, notions of human rights still place the value of society/community over the individual. Biggar, *What's Wrong with Rights?*, 193.

25. Heard from Rabbi L. Kelemen in Jerusalem, 1998.

# CHAPTER ONE

# Self-Endangerment in Medical Experimentation and Modern History

On the wall of the main auditorium in Cedars-Sinai Medical Center in Los Angeles is a mural titled *Jewish Contributions to Medicine*. It depicts thirty-six of the most influential Jewish healers throughout history, beginning with Moses holding the *nachash hanechoshet*, the copper serpent, followed by Mar Shmuel, a leading second-century Babylonian rabbi and the most noted physician of the Talmudic era, and Maimonides, before gradually making its way to the modern era. One of the American figures on the mural, not as well known as he should be, is Dr. Jesse Lazear (the part of that mural depicting Lazear is on the cover of this book).

Dr. Lazear was born in Baltimore, Maryland, in 1866 and earned his undergraduate degree at Johns Hopkins University before completing medical school at the Columbia University College of Physicians and Surgeons. He then undertook specialization training in Paris at the Institut Pasteur. He was married in 1896 and had two children.[1]

In 1898 the Spanish-American War broke out, in which the US Army lost 6,406 troops, 5,438 of whom died from yellow fever. This degree of loss due to contagion was obviously unsustainable for a military and led to public outcries, prompting US Surgeon-General George Miller Sternberg to take action.[2]

One of the most important actions was the formation by the US Army in 1900 of the Yellow Fever Board, which was commanded by US Army physician Walter Reed. The goal of this board was to conduct research to determine how yellow fever is transmitted so that its spread might be prevented. Yellow fever epidemics during the late eighteenth and early nineteenth centuries had created a culture in which solo researchers tried to become heroes to solve the problem. At the beginning of the twentieth century, Lazear was determined to find the cure and become such a hero. At the time, there were numerous theories of how the disease spread, such as by bacteria on clothing, insects, and, more specifically, mosquitoes. Lazear was convinced that the best available evidence suggested a living host for yellow fever, so he pursued the theory of mosquito transmission.

As a result of earlier research scandals, Sternberg had issued strict directives that nobody could be experimented on without consent and that all consent had to be carefully documented. This gave rise to what was known as "the golden rule self-experimentation," which said that researchers were expected not to try anything on others that they wouldn't be willing to try on themselves.[3]

Lazear made significant progress on his theories while conducting research at a hospital in Havana, Cuba. He ruled out a bacterium as the disease agent and eventually confirmed his hypothesis that mosquitoes transmitted this disease by allowing mosquitoes to feed first on patients infected with yellow fever, followed by allowing study volunteers to be bitten by those same mosquitoes, after which many study volunteers eventually fell ill with yellow fever. In this process, his team determined that an infectious particle too small to be filtered with a standard bacterial filter was the source of the disease, thus discovering the first human virus.[4] He wrote to his wife in a letter dated September 8, 1900, "I rather think I am on the track of the real germ."[5]

Given the "golden rule self-experimentation" ethic of the time, Lazear decided to intentionally have himself and two of his research assistants be bitten by contaminated mosquitoes as part of his experiments. The two men Lazear exposed to yellow fever via these mosquitoes recovered. Lazear, however, was not so lucky. He contracted the disease and died two and a half weeks after writing that hopeful letter, just twelve days after being bitten at the age of only thirty-four. The fact that this was a deliberate act, that his infection was the result of self-experimentation, was covered up at the time—for reasons unknown but possibly connected with family insurance policies.[6] The researchers who recovered were awarded Congressional Medals of Honor, and Lazear became known as "the martyr to science," even though the results of his particular self-inflicted bite unfortunately did not assist the research due to lack of documentation. As a result of this episode, Sternberg enacted strict research regulations and forbade any further self-experimentation, fearing that this practice could deplete medical personnel.[7]

Can Lazear's altruism be justified? What does Judaism say about putting oneself at such risk for the sake of the health and safety of the broader society? Although Lazear was a Jew, there is little evidence to suggest that he was observant, and hence he was likely unfamiliar with most Jewish law. But he may have known of Purim, and it is in the biblical book of Esther where significant guidance on navigating this ethical dilemma may be found. Rabbi Joseph B. Soloveitchik, one of the greatest American Talmudists of the twentieth century, argues that there is one verse that is the central *halakhah* (law) of the entire book of Esther (4:16): "And if I perish, I perish." When Esther was asked to risk her life to come to the defense of her people before the king, she did so. According to Rabbi Soloveitchik, this verse thus requires an individual to sacrifice their life if the destiny and future of the community are at stake.[8]

Rabbi Soloveitchik illustrates this principle with a profound episode from Jewish history that may have been forgotten had he not reminded the world of it.[9] It occurred one Hoshanah Rabbah holiday (the holiday that falls at the end of the Sukkot festival) in Vilna during the eighteenth century. An apostate Jew hid a stolen icon from the main cathedral inside the Old Synagogue and brought the archbishop to catch Jews engaging in the ritual pounding of their Hoshanot (willow branches) at the church icon. Of course, the Jews in the synagogue that day had no idea the icon was even there; they had been set up. Nevertheless, thirty members of the Jewish Council (the *parnasim* of the community) were arrested for this "crime" and would certainly be put to death as a result.

Upon hearing of this impending tragedy, a local rabbi named Rav Man ben Rav Man decided that he wanted to take the blame for this action in order to spare his community. Rav Man consulted with the community rabbi, Shmuel Acharon, arguing that he was certain that if he told the authorities that he was the one who stole the icon, they would punish him with death but let the thirty Jews go. Rabbi Shmuel felt that he had to ask the Vilna Gaon this difficult question before giving Rav Man guidance. However, before Rabbi Shmuel could tell Rav Man what to do, Rav Man told him not to ask the leading rabbi of the generation, the Vilna Gaon, because he had already realized what he must do based on the actions of Esther in the Bible.

That night, which was the Shemini Atzeret holiday, the holiday immediately after Sukkot, Rav Man turned himself in to the authorities, and indeed they allowed the other Jews to go free. They began to torture Rav Man and did so for many months until finally executing him publicly in front of the cathedral on the holiday of Shavuot, which is celebrated approximately nine months after Sukkot. We know this story because Rabbi Soloveitchik, when visiting Vilna, heard the E-l Malei Rachamim memorial prayer that was recited in Vilna for Rav Man every Hoshanah Rabbah and Shavuot. Since the destruction of European Jewry during the Holocaust, to the best of my knowledge, this E-l Malei is no longer recited anywhere, yet another tradition lost due to the Holocaust. However, thanks to Rav Soloveitchik, this story and its vital lesson remain.

Perhaps further support for Rav Man's actions can be found in the Talmudic account of the "Harugei Lod," the brothers executed in the city of Lod during the time of the Roman occupation of the Land of Israel. The Roman emperor's daughter was found murdered, and the Jewish community was blamed. The emperor threatened the Jews with mass execution unless they could produce the murderer. To save the Jewish people, two innocent brothers, Lilianus and Pappus, stepped forward and falsely confessed to the crime, and thus only the two of them were executed by the Roman official Turyanus, sparing the rest of the Jewish community.[10] Some rabbinic authorities have thus permitted (but not required) voluntary self-sacrifice in order to rescue the broader community, based on the rabbis' praise for these righteous brothers.[11]

On the other hand, Rabbi Isaac Kook (the first Ashkenazic chief rabbi in pre-state Israel) disagreed, arguing that although saving the broader community is a very high value, and one should engage in small risk to attempt to do so, these stories do not prove that one who is not currently in any danger may opt to risk their life for the sake of the broader community, since the brothers in Lod and Queen Esther would have died along with their community anyway.[12] Indeed, support for this position can be found in the fact that one who has been exiled to a city of refuge may never leave the protection of that city, even if all of Israel needs their help, because doing so would make them vulnerable to being killed.[13] This ruling implies that the community does not necessarily take priority over an individual's life.[14]

In 2020 related questions arose once again, this time in the context of medical experimentation with regard to the coronavirus pandemic. As the death toll climbed, along with the costs of shutting down entire countries to prevent the spread of the virus, there was a mad rush to develop a vaccine. But developing vaccines takes time, in part because of tragic stories such as that of Dr. Lazear. By the end of the twentieth century, very strict governmental protocols and regulations on vaccine testing were developed to try to prevent unnecessary deaths.

One such approach to testing potentially new vaccines is that researchers must randomize test subjects into two groups: Group A gets the vaccine, while Group B gets a placebo. Then the researchers simply wait and see if more people from Group B get sick than do those in Group A, thus demonstrating that the vaccine is effective. However, it can take many months before researchers get their answer because, in its simplest form, this kind of study depends on waiting for people to be naturally exposed to the virus in their everyday lives. When, as part of social efforts to stem the spread of whatever is causing an epidemic people are forced to stay apart—that is, to engage in "social distancing"—it takes even longer to see if a proposed vaccine is effective.

To speed things up, some suggested an alternative protocol called a "challenge study." A challenge study works very similarly to the traditional study described above—some people are given an experimental vaccine, and some are not. However, what differs is that in the challenge study, all study subjects are deliberately exposed to the disease for which the vaccine is being developed. Researchers then compare the two groups—the vaccine versus the control—knowing that everyone was exposed to the disease. Running a study in this manner could save several months (and thus thousands, if not millions, of lives).[15] However, to expose people to a disease that is particularly dangerous, such as coronavirus, makes this a much riskier study. Some may get very sick, and a few may even die.

Based on the opinion of Rabbi Soloveitchik, drawing from the precedent of Queen Esther, I believe the lesson here is that, with proper informed consent, it would certainly be permitted and even a very pious act to serve as a participant in a challenge study associated with rapidly developing a vaccine for a disease such as the coronavirus.[16] Even according to the stricter opinion of Rabbi Kook, mentioned above, for a disease such as the coronavirus, the level of risk for those enrolling in such a study is relatively low (only young, healthy people are accepted for these studies, and they receive careful medical oversight and attention), and because coronavirus put everyone in the world at risk, anyone who might volunteer to be a subject in such a study was already at some risk just by living in society. Entering the study simply allows exposure to happen in a controlled setting, and the results can significantly benefit the entire society, so while not obligatory, this choice could thus be seen as a mitzvah.[17]

Similarly, although neither those entering a challenge study nor Dr. Lazear make their sacrifices only for the Jewish community, and while the various stories of risk that we have discussed in this chapter are certainly not identical, it seems that Dr. Lazear's actions can nonetheless also be justified and deserving of praise because he didn't know for certain that he would die, the results of his risky experiments could potentially save the masses, and he was personally at risk for yellow fever anyway, along with everyone else in society.

May we never again face such dilemmas, but we can take comfort in knowing that from Persia to Vilna to the United States, as life-and-death communal challenges have inevitably arisen, our tradition has provided clear guidance, and in every generation heroic individuals have stepped up to respond to the call of the hour.

# NOTES

1. "Biography of Jesse W. Lazear," *Military Medicine* 166, suppl. 1 (September 2001): 24.

2. Robert Baker, *Before Bioethics: A History of American Medical Ethics from the Colonial Period to the Bioethics Revolution* (New York: Oxford University Press, 2013), 255, 258. Although his name sounds Jewish, the story is told that Frank Heynick, author of *Jews and Medicine: An Epic Saga* (Hoboken, NJ: KTAV, 2003), was disappointed when he came across the name of George Sternberg just as he was completing his manuscript. He had not mentioned Sternberg in his book, and the idea of researching yet another life, editing, and adding to the already six-hundred-page book was disheartening. After further research it turned out that Sternberg was not Jewish—"Thank heavens!" said the ecstatic Heynick. Max Gross, "Doctor Writes 'Epic Saga' of Jews in Medicine," *Jewish Daily Forward*, August 15, 2003.

3. Baker, *Before Bioethics*, 255.

4. "The History of Vaccines," An Educational Resource by the College of Physicians of Philadelphia, n.d., https://www.historyofvaccines.org/content/jesse-lazear.

5. Lawrence K. Altman, *Who Goes First? The Story of Self-Experimentation in Medicine* (Berkeley: University of California Press, 1987), 149–50.

6. Altman writes that the truth was discovered in 1947 by Philip S. Hench from Lazear's own notebook.

7. Baker, *Before Bioethics*, 258.

8. *Mesorat HaRav Megillat Esther* (New York/Jerusalem: Orthodox Union Press, 2017), 93. Rabbi Zilberstein also quotes this verse to support self-endangerment for the sake of attempting to save the masses (*Shiurei Torah LeRofim* 6:396, 316n5). See also Responsa *Shvut Yaakov* 2:117.

9. *Mesorat HaRav Megillat Esther*, 90–93.

10. *Bava Batra* 10b, Rashi, s.v. *harugei Lod*; *Ta'anit* 18b, Rashi, s.v. *beLudkya*. Similarly, perhaps additional support can be brought from the Maharshal, who argues that King Saul killed himself (I Sam. 31:4) because he worried that if the Philistines would have captured and publicly tortured him, many Jews would have died in their attempts to avenge him and save his life, so he killed himself in order to save their lives (*Yam Shel Shlomo*, Bava Kamma, 8:59).

11. *Yeshuot Yaakov*, YD 157:1, available at https://hebrewbooks.org/pdfpager.aspx?req= 9210&st=&pgnum=218&hilite=; see also *Tiferet Yisrael* on *Mishnah Berakhot* 1:3 quoted in *Pitchei Teshuvah*, YD 157(3), which states that one may take on a small degree of risk in order to fulfill a mitzvah, which may even be obligatory if it is for the sake of saving the masses (*hatzalat rabbim*), as quoted in *Mishpat Kohen* 143.

12. On saving the broader community, see detailed discussion on the importance of the entire community in Jewish thought and bioethics, in A. Steinberg, *HaRefuah KeHalakhah*, vol. 5 (Jerusalem, 2017), 107–8. *Mishpat Kohen* 143 argues, based on the *Sifrei* and *Bava Metzia* 112a, that when the danger is distant (*safek rachok*) or a standard level of risk that people generally enter into, then one should do so in order to attempt to save the many, and not worry about oneself, as many great Jews have done throughout history, as long as it is not a certain danger (in which case the obligation of *vechai bahem* takes precedence). He argues in *Mishpat Kohen* 144 (9–10) that there is no obligation for an individual to save the entire

Jewish community since everyone must do their part. He thus suggests that at first Esther thought there were other ways to save the people without her risking her life, until she was convinced that she needed to do it herself. When one does so they get reward and credit for doing a mitzvah, even if it is not obligatory. He concludes that there could be times when a person could determine that they want to surrender their life for the higher value of the community when they calculate that the whole is more valuable than their own life (*Mishpat Kohen*, 15–17). Rabbi Kook's claim that Esther would have died along with the Jewish community is based on Rashi to Esther 4:13, that Mordecai told her she would be included in the decree to kill all the Jews. Rabbi Kook claims that it was only once she found out that she would likely die along with everyone else that she realized she was obligated to take this risk (*Mishpat Kohen* 143). However, the suggestion that Esther would have been killed along with the Jewish community can be challenged and does not seem to be the opinion of Rabbi Soloveitchik or Rav Man, quoted above.

13. *Mishneh Torah, Hilkhot Rotze'ach* 7:8. Based on this, Rabbi Meir Simchah of Dvinsk also seems to be of the opinion that one should never endanger themselves, even in order to save the entire nation (*Meshech Chokhmah, Shemot* 4:19; *Ohr Same'ach, Hilkhot Rotze'ach* 7:8).

14. See detailed discussion in Jonathan Sacks, *Covenant & Conversation, a Weekly Reading of the Jewish Bible: Numbers* (New Milford, CT: Maggid, 2017), 407–17.

15. Nir Eyal, Marc Lipsitch, and Peter G. Smith, "Human Challenge Studies to Accelerate Coronavirus Vaccine Licensure," *Journal of Infectious Diseases* 221, no. 11 (June 2020): 1752–56, https://doi.org/10.1093/infdis/jiaa152; and Andrea Cioffi, "COVID-19: Is Everything Appropriate to Create an Effective Vaccine?" *Journal of Infectious Diseases* (April 29, 2020), https://www.ncbi.nlm.nih.gov/pmc/articles/PMC7197522/. See also Correspondence: "Coronavirus Disease 2019: Is Everything Lawful to Create an Effective Vaccine?" *Journal of Infectious Diseases* (July 1, 2020), https://academic.oup.com/jid/advance-article-pdf/doi/10.1093/infdis/jiaa217/33283826/jiaa217.pdf; and Garth Rapeport, Emma Smith, Anthony Gilbert, Andrew Catchpole, Helen McShane, and Christopher Chiu, "SARS-CoV-2 Human Challenge Studies—Establishing the Model during an Evolving Pandemic," *New England Journal of Medicine* 385 (September 9, 2021): 961–64, http://dx.doi.org/10.1056/NEJMp2106970. A full book was published on the ethics of challenge studies: Euzebiusz Jamrozik and Michael J. Selgelid, *Human Challenge Studies in Endemic Settings: Ethical and Regulatory Issues* (Cham: Springer International, 2021); on Jewish perspectives, see Sharon Galper Grossman and Shamai Grossman, "Signing Up for a COVID-19 Vaccine Trial," *LehrHaus*, August 18, 2020, https://thelehrhaus.com/timely-thoughts/signing-up-for-a-covid-19-vaccine-trial/#_edn1.

16. See note 12 above, *Lev Avraham*, 284, and extensive discussion in Steinberg, *HaRefuah KeHalakhah*, 53, on risk and entering experimental studies in Jewish law.

17. Indeed, after I wrote this chapter, Rabbi A. Weiss wrote a responsum to this author, published in Responsa *Minchat Asher—Magefat HaKorona*, 8(2), in which he agreed that entering such a study is a *mitzvah gedolah* and *pikuach nefesh* because there is a high chance that it could save an entire generation from illness and death. Rabbi Weiss argues that risk and self-endangerment are permissible when it is for essential public benefit, especially when it is young and healthy people acting on behalf of crucial communal needs. He also quotes

Rabbi S. Z. Auerbach, who notes that just as when there is a military threat to a community, leaders can endanger soldiers' lives by sending them to war for the good of the nation, so too the need to test medicines can be justified as a mitzvah war of saving lives and protecting the community. Responsa *Minchat Shlomo* 2:82(12); see also Rabbi S. Yisraeli in *Amud HaYemini* (Jerusalem, 2000), 17.

# CHAPTER TWO

# Allocation and Distribution of Scarce Resources

Having discussed expectations of risk for others, we now turn our attention to a complicated caveat: what to do when we are simply incapable of helping everyone equally? Many lessons have been learned during the COVID-19 pandemic, when many health care systems faced severe shortages, significantly affecting clinical decision-making for physicians, patients, and families. Shortages of ICU beds and ventilators have created very real concerns about how to properly ration them, which leads to wrenching life-and-death decisions. Triage priority decisions also have to be made about allocating limited amounts of medications, tests, and vaccines. The principles and my suggestions discussed in this chapter are relevant not only to such pandemic situations but can be applied to many areas of medical triage and rationing, such as natural disasters, mass casualty events, war, surges of patients, and shortages of equipment or staff.[1]

There are many approaches to the most efficient and ethical allocation of scarce resources in the contemporary secular bioethics literature.[2] Some approaches focus on equality and thus favor lotteries or first come, first served. Others simply favor younger patients who have had the least amount of life to live, while others give treatment priority and the most attention to the sickest patients and those who are at highest risk of immediate death. However, most approaches focus instead on how to save the maximum number of lives. But how to do so is often not easy to determine.

Hospitals typically develop their own triage policies in the event of scarce medical resources, guided by governmental agencies. The process of creating such policies often also involves a bioethics committee and approval by medical

staff leadership. An allocation review committee and specific critical care allocation teams then implement the policies in each case that arises, frequently using algorithms to determine and rank these priorities of need for each patient.[3]

What becomes most complex and controversial is that, when all clinical determination metrics are equal, many of the tie-breaking triage decisions become
completely value based. It is at this point that religious traditions and spiritual
leaders can provide significant input to policy development. Furthermore, for
religious health care providers and patients who would like treatment decisions
to be made based on their own values as much as possible, spiritual care providers can be influential in guiding the implementation of religiously sensitive
medical decision-making.

Indeed, Judaism provides detailed guidance for all areas of life, including
times of crisis. This rich tradition is especially important in considering unique
approaches that may become necessary during challenging times. It is therefore
beneficial to examine some of the key Jewish values that arise in this context,
which are summarized below.

## SUMMARY OF SOME JEWISH EMERGENCY TRIAGE VALUES

1. Triage as much as possible to try to avoid the need to withdraw any treatments.

   - The goal is always to save as many people as possible.
   - Prioritize patients who are most likely to benefit and who have overall
     better chances of survival.
   - Prioritize patients with the potential to live a full lifespan over those
     who are terminal.
   - Base decisions only on the clinically relevant health of the patient, not
     their socioeconomic status, race, gender, and so on.

2. If a patient will likely not survive and other patients need their room, ventilator, staff, or other resources, it is preferable to withhold further interventions from that patient in order to allow them to die naturally rather than by
   withdrawing any interventions.

3. If there is no other choice and it seems clear that a patient currently on a
   respirator will die soon in any case, withdrawal of a respirator can only be
   considered on a case-by-case basis, in consultation with a *posek* (senior rabbinic authority in Jewish law).

## DETAILED DISCUSSION

Below is a more detailed discussion to more explicitly articulate and clarify the underlying values that provide the foundation for the above framework. The primary goals are to save as many people as possible and do so by prioritizing according to clear and transparent principles based in classical Jewish sources and the works of contemporary rabbinic scholars.

### Saving the Many

A fundamental principle of triage in Jewish law is that priority must be given to saving as many people as possible.[4] This is based on a classic rabbinic concept known as *hatzalat rabim* (saving the many).[5] For this reason, rabbinic authorities encourage an approach to triage that bypasses treating those who are too sick to benefit from, or too well to absolutely need, treatment. Their reasoning is that since treating these patients requires more time and resources, many others will die waiting. Treating the more moderately ill should be the focus of efforts since that generally takes less time and uses fewer intensive resources, thus enabling treatment of more people.[6] In the context of the COVID-19 pandemic, when vaccines were first made available but there was not yet enough for everyone, some also suggested that this principle may give priority access to vaccines to the potential biggest spreaders of the virus ("super spreaders").[7]

### Priorities

Some of the following relevant priorities for various triage circumstances are detailed in Jewish law:

- *Chances and certainty*: The key principle of all triage decisions is the medical likelihood of success of treatment, determined by prioritizing treating the patients with the greatest chances of survival.[8] Additionally, in Jewish law, a definite danger takes precedence over an uncertain danger.[9] Therefore, in a situation in which one patient can certainly or likely be saved and the outcome for the other patient is uncertain, priority must be given to the person who has better chances of being saved.[10]
- *Potential for full life*: Similarly, when two patients are waiting for a ventilator or medication but only enough for one is available, if one patient has the potential to live a full lifespan after being placed on the ventilator or treated and the other is terminal, Jewish law prioritizes the patient who is more likely to live a full lifespan.[11]

- *Individuals needed by society*: Although great care should be taken to treat all people equally, with no priority based on socioeconomic status, race, gender, and so on, an individual who is desperately needed by society, such as frontline health care providers (particularly when they are also at high risk of infection) or those deemed essential to society, may sometimes gain priority if absolutely necessary, when all other factors are equal.[12]

- *Preference to withhold rather than withdraw*: If a ventilator, dialysis machine, or other mechanical life-sustaining device of a patient who is completely dependent on it will be needed eventually by another patient, it is preferable to allow the former to die naturally through passive means, such as not refilling IV medication bags or not increasing ventilator settings, rather than by terminal extubation.[13] This approach may sometimes include allowing patients with very low chances of survival to be given Do Not Resuscitate status, which will make their ventilator available after the patient dies naturally.[14] Furthermore, it is not always required to intubate (put on a respirator) a dying patient who is suffering, particularly in triage situations when other patients may be able to benefit more from the limited respirators available, even if those other patients are not yet present in the hospital but are expected.[15]

  This preference is not only due to religious perspectives that differentiate between the morality of withholding versus withdrawing life-sustaining treatments but also is an attempt to mitigate some of the anguish that clinicians often experience when asked to withdraw ventilators for reasons other than the welfare of the patient.[16]

- *Situations in which treatment was already initiated*: Ideally, a patient who is already intubated or being treated, even if not likely to survive, acquires a certain right to continued treatment. It follows that, whenever possible, treatment should not be removed from one patient in order to treat another.[17] However, a patient who is terminal or has a very low likelihood of recovery may be moved out of the emergency room or intensive care unit in order to make room for a patient who is likely to benefit more from that higher level of treatment, provided that nothing is done to actively shorten the terminal patient's life.[18]

- *Someone who will die immediately*: If there is a choice of which patient to extubate, it is ideal not to extubate someone who will die immediately as a result and instead choose someone who may be able to breathe on their own for some time after they are extubated.[19]

Under normal circumstances, terminal extubation (removing a patient from a ventilator that is sustaining their life) is forbidden by most rabbinic authorities.[20] However, there is a minority opinion based on the ruling of Rabbi Moshe Isserles (Code of Jewish Law YD 339:1) that one may actively remove an external impediment to death of a patient who is already almost certainly in the process of dying imminently (*gosses*).[21] Some rule that a ventilator can be categorized as an artificial impediment to dying since it mechanically prevents the soul from departing. Thus, it is not only permitted to remove a ventilator from a dying patient but it may even be required to do so to relieve suffering.[22] Since there are conflicting opinions on this matter, and some argue that deactivating a ventilator of a patient who is dependent on it falls under the severe prohibition of murder, many conclude that we must be strict and forbid deactivation of a ventilator at the end of life.[23] However, in a difficult situation in which there is a severe shortage of ventilators, and the purpose of removing one patient from a ventilator is to save another patient's life, there may be a stronger basis to permit doing so, particularly in some cases of dying patients who have no chance of recovery.[24]

This approach can reduce suffering and enable the saving of many lives.[25] Although saving one or even many lives does not override active killing in Jewish law, this *hatzalat rabim* perspective favors the position that terminal extubation is not always viewed as *killing* but may be seen as allowing to die or failing to save, which can be permitted for a dying patient.[26] However, terminal extubation can be permitted only on a case-by-case basis after careful review and determination that there is no other option, such as those detailed above.

## CONCLUSION

This chapter is not meant to imply that Jewish patients should be treated differently from others, but it is intended to serve as a guide to decision-making based on Jewish values. In an emergency situation, frontline medical professionals must make urgent and difficult choices. Rabbis cannot be present for every such decision, nor is there time to deliberate whether rabbis support each decision. Accordingly, it would be prudent for rabbinic authorities to take part in creating triage decision-making processes in order to ensure that the most appropriate approach is considered, whenever possible.

Some health care providers might debate the logic of these rulings, but they are based on profound wisdom and tradition. These excruciating decisions can induce severe moral distress. The more that we can do to help people make them in accordance with ancient but relevant religious teachings and wisdom, the more we can prevent some of the moral distress associated with such crises and maintain our own ethical integrity and our relationships with God. And of course, when engaging in such difficult dilemmas, it becomes especially important to care for the emotional and spiritual well-being of medical professionals, patients, and their families not only so that patients can survive physically but also so that they and their caregivers may survive as "whole" as possible.

Discussion of allocation of limited resources leads to fundamental questions about the ideals of a moral society, individual rights to health care, and government and societal obligations to provide it for all. We will thus now turn our attention to an analysis of Jewish wisdom and precedent as it relates to the highly contentious and ever relevant issue of societal obligations to provide universal access to health care.

# NOTES

1. On the different uses and meanings of the words "triage" and "rationing" in modern medicine, see Tom L. Beauchamp and James F. Childress, *Principles of Biomedical Ethics*, 8th ed. (New York: Oxford University Press, 2019), 304–12. "Triage," which refers to the urgent process of screening patients, is also different from "allocation," which refers to the ways in which resources are distributed. See *Encyclopedia of Bioethics*, 4th ed. (Macmillan Reference, 2014), 3108.

2. See review in Govind Persad, Alan Wertheimer, and Ezekiel J. Emanuel, "Principles for Allocation of Scarce Medical Interventions," *Lancet* 373, no. 9661 (January 31, 2009): 423–31.

3. See, for example, the California state guidelines: "California SARS-CoV-2 Pandemic Crisis Care Guidelines: Concept of Operations Health Care Facility Surge Operations and Crisis Care," June 2020, https://www.cdph.ca.gov/Programs/CID/DCDC/CDPH%20 Document%20Library/COVID-19/California%20SARS-CoV-2%20Crisis%20Care%20 Guidelines%20-June%208%202020.pdf?eType=EmailBlastContenteId=b2a40a32-36f8-4 7d5-b0f3-4412e7c47e12.

4. Indeed, some have argued that when there are many patients in need, all arriving simultaneously, and when there are insufficient resources to treat all of them at that time, this approach of prioritizing the moderately injured (ignoring the severe and minor injuries) so the greatest number of lives can be saved is the ideal approach ethically and halakhically. A. Steinberg, *HaRefuah Ke-Halakhah*, vol. 1 (Jerusalem: printed by the author, 2017), 5, 82. However, in using this approach, the medical professionals must be careful to frequently reevaluate the patients who are awaiting treatment since their conditions may change, as may the staff availabilities. This approach is virtually identical to that most frequently advocated by secular bioethicists as well. Ezekiel J. Emanuel, Govind Persad, Ross Upshur, Beatriz Thome, Michael Parker, Aaron Glickman, Cathy Zhang, Connor Boyle, Maxwell Smith, and James P. Phillips, "Fair Allocation of Scarce Medical Resources in the Time of Covid-19," *New England Journal of Medicine* 382, no. 21 (May 2020): 2052.

5. Rabbi Zilberstein, (*Shiurei Torah LeRofim* 3:161) bases this primarily on the ruling of the

*Chazon Ish* (*Sanhedrin* 25 and YD 69) that if an arrow is shot in a way that it could kill many people but it can be diverted in a way that will kill just one person, that should be done in order to save the many.

6. Responsa *Minchat Asher* 1:115, 2:126; and *Shiurei Torah LeRofim* 3:161, 66–67, 73. Rabbi Zilberstein has approved of health care professionals abandoning a patient who is not certainly salvageable, even if they have already begun treating him or her, in order to save many who are certainly salvageable since abandoning one patient need not be seen as an act of murder but as an act of saving life. However, this must be a situation in which the medic is simply allowing the patient to die in order to save the many but not actually performing an action that causes the patient's death. However, even if a medic did so, it would not be classified as murder since it is done in the context of lifesaving (69–70).

7. In an unpublished responsum to this author, Rabbi Y. T. Rimon suggested that perhaps society would benefit the most if those who are younger and interacting with more people, and thus most likely to spread the virus, are vaccinated first. This approach has also been advocated by some bioethicists and public health professionals. See Dana Goldman, David Conti, and Matthew Kahn, "The COVID-19 Vaccine Model Needs to Prioritize 'Superspreaders.' Here Is Why," Leonard D. Schaeffer Center for Health Policy & Economics, September 3, 2020, https://healthpolicy.usc.edu/article/covid-19-vaccine-model -needs-to-prioritize-superspreaders-here-is-why/. However, Rabbi Rimon concludes that Jewish law prioritizes saving life that is in immediate danger (based on *Noda BeYehudah*, YD 210), and thus those who are in greater danger should be vaccinated first.

8. *Minchat Asher—Magefat HaKorona*, 7. These principles (prioritize individuals in greatest danger who have the highest need and there is the greater likelihood of the treatment being effective) apply equally to ventilator triage and vaccine triage (*Minchat Asher—Magefat HaKorona*, 151). Likelihood of success is also a key criterion in secular bioethics; see Beauchamp and Childress, *Principles of Biomedical Ethics*, 309.

9. *Nishmat Avraham*, YD 252:8(2) (319 in 3rd ed.), based on *Pri Megadim* 328:47(1); *Tzitz Eliezer* 9:17 (10:5) and 28:3. High risk of infection is the reason individuals living in nursing homes and long-term care facilities were prioritized to receive the vaccine. The CDC also prioritized those with social or communal vulnerabilities to receive the vaccine. Halakhic approaches only consider the level of medical need, not social considerations, but some have suggested that vulnerability can be taken into account based on the ruling of the *Shulchan Arukh* (YD 252:1) that ransoming a captive precedes feeding or clothing the poor. See discussion in Jonathan K. Crane, "Jewish Ethics in COVID-19," *Journal of Jewish Ethics* 6, no. 1 (2020): 21. Others have suggested that because people of color and those of lower socioeconomic status often suffer from more chronic health conditions and are victims of disparities in health care, they are thus at more risk of serious illness, so Jewish law may give them some priority. Alan Jotkowitz, "Triage during the Covid-19 Pandemic: A Halakhic Perspective," *Hakira* 29 (Winter 2021): 140.

10. *Iggerot Moshe*, CM 2:73(2); Responsa *Minchat Shlomo* 2:86(2); Responsa *Shevet HaLevi* 10:167; *Kovetz Teshuvot* 3:159; Responsa *Minchat Asher* 2:126. Rabbi Zilberstein, *Shiurei Torah Le-Rofim* 3:161, 67, bases this on *Mishnah Berurah* 334:68, which rules that if two people are in a burning house, one healthy, the other in life-threatening danger, and both cannot be saved,

one should save the healthy person first, since the other one is not certainly salvageable (although others disagree with this proof; see Responsa *Shvivei Aish*, YD 2:394). When it comes to vaccine triage, this value might give priority to those who have not had the illness over those who had already been afflicted with the illness and recovered since they might already have antibodies and may not benefit from the vaccine as much as those who have not had the illness. Rabbi Dr. Aaron E. Glatt, "Who Should Get the Covid 19 Vaccine First," YouTube, December 31, 2020, https://youtu.be/NhKdmk2h-wo.

11. If a terminal patient is currently in need of limited medical resources but there is a strong likelihood that a patient who can still live a full lifespan may arrive in need of this treatment at any time, many leading authorities argue that one who has a chance for a full lifespan still takes priority over the one who is terminal. The hospital thus has the right to designate its devices only for such patients who may arrive, even though the patient who can live a full lifespan is not actually present at the time (*Teshuvot VeHanhagot* 1:858; *Tzitz Eliezer* 17:72; Responsa *Minchat Shlomo, Tinyana* 2–3:86:11; *HaRefuah KeHalakhah* 5, 85–86). On the other hand, some argue that since we currently have no obligation to save anyone else who is not in our presence, we should give preference to the terminal patient who is present and in immediate need, even if the goal is simply to relieve suffering and not save a life, unless perhaps if the patient with the better likelihood of survival is already en route to the hospital (Responsa *Shevet HaLevi* 6:242; *Shiurei Torah LeRofim* 3:164, 93, 96, 103–4). Along similar lines, Rabbi M. Feinstein rules that in triage situations, when all else is equal, patients should be treated based on a first come, first served basis (*Iggerot Moshe*, CM 2:74). Indeed, his son-in-law, Rabbi Tendler, reports that when Rabbi Feinstein was asked by the chief rabbi of Israel who should be prioritized to receive the very limited penicillin available in Israel at the time, Rabbi Feinstein answered that it should be given to the first patient the physician saw who needed the medication (*Sefer Kavod HaRav*, 169). Rabbi A. Weiss has expressed disagreement with this approach (*Minchat Asher–Magefat HaKorona*, 7). Many rabbinic authorities rule that anyone who will not survive for more than twelve months is considered "terminal" (*Nishmat Avraham*, YD 155 [84–85 in 3rd ed.]), whereas others argue that six months is a more precise definition of "terminal" (Responsa *Minchat Asher* 1:115[2]). Prioritizing the patient who is more likely to live a full lifespan is based on the concept that "we are not concerned with the value of temporal life (*chayei sha'ah*)" (*Avodah Zarah* 27b), and the ruling of Rabbi Akiva that "your life takes precedence over the life of the other" (*Bava Metzia* 62a). See *Iggerot Moshe*, CM 2:73(2) and 75(2); Responsa *Minchat Shlomo* 86:60; Responsa *Minchat Asher* 1:115(2) and 2:126; and J. David Bleich, "Coronavirus Queries (4): Assignment of Ventilators," *Tradition* 54, no. 1 (Winter 2022). Although since many categorize extubation as killing, one cannot remove from a ventilator a patient who can live only *chayei sha'ah* for the sake of one who can live *chayei olam*. *Iggerot Moshe*, CM 2:73(2); and *Teshuvot VeHanhagot* 1:858. Age should not be a factor; patients should be treated equally regardless of whether one is very elderly or very young, although one who can live longer than a year takes precedence, regardless of how much longer than a year one can live (*Iggerot Moshe*, CM 2:75[2, 7]). However, when it comes to triaging a COVID vaccine, many bioethicists suggest prioritizing older adults because they are at a higher level of risk of death, whereas when it comes to ventilator triage, they prioritize younger, healthier people since the goal in both cases is to maximize

benefit and save as many lives as possible. Emanuel et al., "Fair Allocation of Scarce Medical Resources," 2053; and Nancy S. Jecker, Aaron G. Wightman, and Douglas S. Diekema, "Vaccine Ethics: An Ethical Framework for Global Distribution of COVID-19 Vaccines," *Journal of Medical Ethics* (February 2021): 3. For a different perspective on taking the age of a patient into account in classical Jewish sources, see Dovid Lichtenstein, *Headlines 3* (Cambridge, MA: Shikey, 2022), 48–50.

12. The ranking of priorities detailed in the Mishnah in *Horayot* (3:8) is not generally followed today because they would be very difficult to put into practice and other priorities carry more weight. *Iggerot Moshe*, CM 2:75(7); *Masorat Moshe*, 1:489; Responsa *Minchat Shlomo* 2:86[1]; Steinberg, *HaRefuah KeHalakhah* 5, 80, 88; see also detailed discussion in David Etengoff, "Triage in Halacha: The Threat of an Avian Flu Epidemic," *Journal of Halacha and Contemporary Society* 55 (2008): 84–90. This is because we do not always know how to properly make these determinations today (see *Tzitz Eliezer* 18:1 and 69[1]), or because that *mishnah* refers only to charity distribution (*Meiri* on *Horayot* 3:8, see discussion in Lichtenstein, *Headlines 3*, 53–55), or because those priorities don't apply when people have paid for health care services (*Shiurei Torah LeRofim* 6:401, 333–36). See extensive discussion in Alan Jotkowitz, "A Man Takes Precedence over a Woman When It Comes to Saving a Life," *Tradition* 47, no. 1 (2014): 48–68. Rabbi Zilberstein rules that all people should be treated equally, based only on clinically relevant information and triage protocols, not things like lifestyle or vaccination status, so even a terrorist whose action caused the triage situation must receive the same prioritization as the victims (*Shiurei Torah LeRofim* 6:425, 416). Ability to pay may not be a factor either (Responsa *Minchat Asher* 2:126). The triage protocols adopted by the Israeli Ministry of Health in May 2020 during the COVID-19 pandemic stated that "health care professionals, even if infected while treating COVID-19 patients, will not be given priority unless it is necessary to overcome staff shortages, either by facilitating return to work after their recovery or as an incentive to volunteering. When there is medical equality between two patients, health care professionals will receive priority." "Position Paper: Triage Decisions for Severely Ill Patients during the COVID-19 Pandemic," Joint Commission for the Israel National Council on Bioethics, the Ethics Bureau of the Israel Medical Association and the Israeli Ministry of Health, May 2020, https://www.health.gov.il/Publications Files/position-paper-230520.pdf. Support for an approach that gives priority to health care professionals and those who can save others can be found in the Talmud (*Horayot* 13a), which states that when saving a life, precedence should be given to a *kohen* who is anointed for battle over another *kohen* since the masses are dependent on him; see Rashi there, s.v. *lehachayoto*. Regarding vaccine triage, preference was given for frontline health care providers even though not all agreed that this should be the case regarding ventilator triage, both because of the instrumental value they play in society and pandemic response and because they were considered to be at the highest risk. Emanuel et al., "Fair Allocation of Scarce Medical Resources," 2053. *Shiurei Torah LeRofim* 3:161, 66–67, 73, and 6:425(4), 421, and 6:429, 433. See also Rambam, *Perush Mishnayot* on *Horayot* 3:8. Rabbi Zilberstein compares this to the option to save one boat when two are sinking, in which case the boat with more passengers on board should be saved. Rabbi Zilberstein also argues that an individual who is needed by the community can be compared to "many" and may thus take precedence over another individual

in some cases. Yitzchok Zilberstein (*Shiurei Torah Le-Rofim* 3:161, 52, 66–67, 73; 6:425(4), 421; and 6:429, 433). See also *Tzitz Eliezer* 10, 25:7(12); Steinberg, *HaRefuah KeHalakhah* 5, 90; and Aryeh Dienstag, "Rationing during a Pandemic Flu," *Verapo Yerape* 2 (2010): 181. Many secular bioethicists also support taking an individual's social utility into account; see Beauchamp and Childress, *Principles of Biomedical Ethics*, 311–12. However, in a public teleconference on this topic hosted by Agudas Yisroel on April 6, 2020, Rabbi A. Weiss expressed disagreement with this priority because it is too difficult to accurately determine who is more important to the community.

13. Some authorities rule that vasopressor medications ("pressers" for maintaining blood pressure), such as dopamine, may be withheld from a dying patient who is suffering (but not actively withdrawn, especially if it may lead to an immediate drop in blood pressure and death) by simply refraining from restarting the treatment once the infusion pouch has emptied on its own because this can be considered a medical therapy and not a basic need, such as nutrition or oxygen. Prof. A. Steinberg in the name of Rabbi Auerbach and Rabbi Wosner, *Assia* 63/64, no. 5729: 18–19; and "The Halachic Basis of the Dying Patient Law," *Assia* 6, no. 2 (2008): 30–40, reprinted in *Jewish Medical Ethics*, 3:419. Similarly, Rabbi M. Feinstein has been quoted as ruling that a dying patient who is on a respirator does not need to be given medications to extend his life. Rabbi Aharon Felder, *Rishumei Aharon*, vol. 1, 70 (New York: printed by the author, 2010). This is different from the approach of many secular bioethicists, who advocate actively removing patients from ventilators to make them available for other patients. Emanuel et al., "Fair Allocation of Scarce Medical Resources," 2052.

14. Responsa of Rabbi H. Schachter. Additional concerns related to COVID include the danger that resuscitative efforts cause to medical staff as well as the utilization of very scarce resources, including staff time and protective equipment.

15. *Nishmat Avraham*, YD 339:1(4) (502–6 in 3rd ed.); and *Minchat Asher–Magefat HaKorona*, 7. See also discussion in note 11 above.

16. Robert D. Truog, Christine Mitchell, and George Q. Daley, "The Toughest Triage: Allocating Ventilators in a Pandemic," *New England Journal of Medicine* 382 (May 2020): 1973–75, http://dx.doi.org/10.1056/NEJMp2005689.

17. *Iggerot Moshe*, CM 2:73(2); and Steinberg, *HaRefuah KeHalakhah* 5, 84. *Nishmat Avraham*, YD 252:8(2) (319 in 3rd ed.), quoting Rabbi S. Z. Auerbach and Rabbi A. Weiss (Responsa *Minchat Asher* 1:115[4]), argues that this is not because one has been granted a right to the continued treatment but rather because of the Talmudic ethical principle that we may never sacrifice one life for another, "*ein dochin nefesh mipnei nefesh.*" Similarly, Rabbi Zilberstein (*Shiurei Torah LeRofim* 3:161, 67, 102) argues that a medic who is working on one patient cannot leave that patient for the sake of another because of the principle that one currently involved in performing a mitzvah may not leave it in order to perform another mitzvah, "*osek bemitzvah patur min hamitzvah.*" This remains true even when the second mitzvah opportunity involves a bigger mitzvah (*mitzvah chamurah*) and one is currently engaged in only a smaller mitzvah (*mitzvah kallah*), unless one can do more mitzvot (i.e., save many lives) by abandoning the first patient. In the latter case, one patient can be left behind to save the many (*Shiurei Torah LeRofim*, 73). However, as stated above, one may not do anything to cause

the patient who is being abandoned to die, unless saving the other is more certain (*Shiurei Torah LeRofim*, 73). However, Rabbi Z. N. Goldberg has ruled that the principle that one currently involved in performing a mitzvah may not leave that mitzvah in order to perform another mitzvah (*osek bemitzvah patur min hamitzvah*) should not be applied to this case and that one should indeed abandon the terminal patient in favor of one who arrives later but can potentially live a full lifespan, unless halting interventions for the terminal patient will cause immediate death. "Hafsakat Tipul BeGosses Leshem Hatzalat Choleh Acher," *Techumin* 36, 209–13; and Steinberg, *HaRefuah KeHalakhah* 5, 84–85.

18. Responsa *Minchat Asher* 1:115(4).

19. Rabbi Z. N. Goldberg, in the citation in footnote 22 below, points out that if a patient was to die immediately upon extubation, that cannot be seen merely as "allowing to die" but as causing to die. *Lev Avraham* 32:9 reports that Rabbi S. Z. Auerbach ruled that the patient must be able to survive for at least forty-eight hours, whereas according to Professor Steinberg (personal communication and *Encyclopedia Hilkhatit Refu'it*, 5, 145), also in the name of Rabbi Auerbach, there is no set time period; even a few hours can be enough to determine if the patient was clinically stable enough for withdrawal. (Rabbi A. Weiss, in a personal communication, concurred with this second approach.) Furthermore, even according to some authorities who do not accept brain death as the halakhic definition of death, if the patient is brain dead, the ventilator may be viewed as an impediment that may be removed. For example, Rabbi O. Yosef ruled that a ventilator may be turned off for a brain-dead patient if the family members consent, as long as it can be done without moving the body of the patient (*Shulchan Yosef* 193). Rabbi S. Z. Auerbach also seems to permit extubation once a patient is brain dead because he assumes that a brain-dead patient with no spontaneous respiration can be considered a *gosses*. Responsa *Minchat Shlomo, Tinyana* 2–3:86; *Assia* 53–54 [5754], 5–16, #6–8. This ruling is also recorded in *Nishmat Avraham*, YD 339 (550–51 in 3rd ed.), where Rabbi Auerbach adds that this is not permitted for the sake of organ donation until the patient's heart stops and doctors have waited at least thirty seconds.

20. *Tzitz Eliezer* 17:72(13); and *Iggerot Moshe*, YD 3:132.

21. The Rema prohibits removing a pillow or cushion from under a dying patient because it is said that the feathers of certain fowl cause a prolongation of dying, but he permits removing salt from the patient's tongue that is preventing their soul from leaving them. Some explain that the problem with moving the feathers is that it would involve significant moving of the dying patient (unlike the minor touch involved with removing salt from the tongue), and these movements could lead to the frail patient's death (*Taz*, YD 339:2; and *Shakh*, YD 339:7).

22. Rabbi Z. N. Goldberg permits actively removing a ventilator from a suffering terminal patient if their death is preferable to life (or for one who has no purpose left in their life because of complete lack of comprehension), but only if it does not directly cause the patient to die right away, in which case removing a ventilator would not be seen simply as removing an impediment but rather as a forbidden act of killing the patient. Rabbi Goldberg bases his opinion on the claim that the person is dying of their own underlying illness, and we are not obligated to "not stand idly by" in the case of a *gosses* unless one benefits more from continued life than death. Rabbi Goldberg argues that a person in excruciating pain

may have no will to live on, and while the prohibition against murder would be violated by an "indirect cause" (*grama*), simply removing an object that can save a person, such that the patient does not die as a result of one's action but because of their own underlying illness, is not considered even an "indirect cause." It is thus not forbidden for a suffering dying patient who would prefer death to life. *Moriah* 4–5:88–89 (Elul 5738), 48–56. See also the somewhat similar perspective recorded in the name of Rabbi Moshe Feinstein in *Masorat Moshe*, 4:309–10. Similarly, Rabbi C. D. HaLevi (*Techumin* 2 [5741]: 304; and *Aseh Lekha Rav* 5:29–30) argues that removing a ventilator parallels the Rema's permission to remove salt from a dying patient's tongue. The salt is also put on the tongue with the hope of prolonging life (according to *Beit Lechem Yehudah*), but now that the patient is in the dying process and the salt is only prolonging their suffering, it is an impediment that may be removed to allow the soul to depart (as the experience of the soul trying to leave the body is considered spiritually painful) since there is no prohibition of "do not stand idly by" for a person who is already a *gosses*. For other similar rulings, see Rabbi M. Klein, *Mishneh Halakhot* 7:287; Rabbi B. Rabinowitz, "Symposium on Establishing the Moment of Death and Organ Donation," *Assia* 1 (5736): 197–98; Rabbi S. Goren, *Me'orot* 2 (5740): 28; and Rabbi P. Toledano, *Barkai* 4 (5747): 53–59. On the pain caused to a dying patient's soul by prolonging their life, see *Iggerot Moshe*, YD 2:174 and CM 2:74.

23. *BeMareh HaBazak* 8:39n35; and Rabbi M. Hershler, "*Chiyuv Hatzalah BeCholim UMesukanim*," in *Halakhah URefuah*, 2(33). See also *Nishmat Avraham*, YD 339(2) (552 in 3rd ed.).

24. Rabbi S. Z. Auerbach seems to support an approach similar to that of his son-in-law, Rabbi Z. N. Goldberg (quoted in note 22 above), in a triage situation. Rabbi Auerbach writes that "regarding a ventilator, it depends on the medical considerations, and if in most cases the ventilator would no longer serve a purpose, it is better to remove it so it can be used by another." This is quoted in full in *Assia* 59–60, 15(3–4) (Iyar 5757); see also Steinberg, *HaRefuah KeHalakhah* 6, 359n16 (5, 84 in expanded edition) as well as discussion of this ruling in Jotkowitz, "Triage during the Covid-19 Pandemic," 134–35. Similarly, in a public teleconference on this topic hosted by Agudas Yisroel on April 6, 2020 (https://player.vimeo.com/video/404795764), Rabbi A. Weiss stated that a patient who is already on a respirator may never be extubated for the sake of another patient, even if the other patient has better chances of survival, but "sometimes people are on ventilators and we know that there is no chance of a recovery. It's just keeping them breathing, or not really breathing but pumping air into their lungs until God will decide ultimately to take them home. Some of these people by medical definition might be brain dead, but we do not accept the determination of brain death; therefore we keep them on ventilators. So in that case if there is a patient before us and we could save his life, then that needs a special *sheilas chochom*." He cautioned that this ruling is not definitive, but a rabbi should be asked and it can be dealt with on a case-by-case basis. On the other hand, many rabbinic authorities never permit terminal extubation. For example, Rabbi H. Schachter wrote a responsum during the COVID-19 pandemic that even during such an emergency situation, one may never remove a patient from a respirator if they will die as a result because doing so would be considered murder (see https://7d4ab068-0603-408d-89df-fac4580e17c4.filesusr.com

/ugd/8b9b1c_c43ae9f486e34ee88578fc8004107114.pdf). See also Bleich, "Coronavirus Queries (4): Assignment of Ventilators."

25. A key principle of Jewish medical ethics is that while we try to prolong life and never do anything to hasten a patient's death, we also do not want to prolong a life of pain and suffering. *Iggerot Moshe*, CM 2:73(1). This approach may allow patients in the dying process to die comfortably rather than have their death prolonged. In addition to making ventilators available for patients who need them, this approach may also encourage giving very sick patients a chance to live who would otherwise not have been intubated in the first place out of fear that they would become vent dependent and no rabbi would permit extubation. Rabbis sometimes discourage intubation for patients with a very low likelihood of recovery so that the patient doesn't become stuck on the ventilator indefinitely, thus severely prolonging their pain and dying process. However, if a rabbi or doctor knows that a patient can be extubated if the ventilator is not effective for them, then perhaps there is more likelihood that they would be willing to give such patients a chance to try the ventilator, and sometimes it may be effective and save the patient's life.

26. Rema, YD 157:1. On the other hand, the *Talmud Yerushalmi* (*Terumot* 8:12) suggests that someone who deserves to die, like Sheva ben Bikhri, may be handed over in order to save the masses. Rambam, *Yesodei HaTorah* 5:5. See also note 22 above.

# CHAPTER THREE

# Universal Health Care

The question of the "right" to fair, universal, and comprehensive health care has been debated for quite a while, but rapid expansion of modern medical technology has led to this becoming a perennial issue that impacts a tremendous number of people. Controlling rising costs, determining priorities, and ensuring fair distribution and access to health care are central questions now that medicine can accomplish so much, is so expensive, and provides so many treatment options.[1]

In the past—and even today, in many poor and developing countries—there was no formalized health care system, and people simply paid out of pocket when they needed medical attention, if they could afford it. However, in the twentieth century, many countries have decided that society has an interest in providing the best possible health care system in order to keep all of its citizens healthy, treat them when they are sick, and help people avoid financial devastation due to medical costs. There are many models that various countries have implemented in order to try to achieve these outcomes. Some have determined that it is the obligation of the government to finance health care, supported by taxes, both as a public service and as a human right. In such a system health care is provided to everyone, much like libraries or the fire department. Other models seek to provide universal access but also limit the role of the government by creating a health insurance system that is paid for jointly by employers and employees. These models sometimes also include government-run insurance options, which often provide more benefits to those who can contribute financially. Others prefer a completely free market system of health care to prevent government intervention or monopolies and to increase efficiency, quality, and innovation. There are many variations and strategies, and each has its own benefits and shortcomings. It is crucial to clearly articulate the underlying goals and ideology of any given communal health care provision system to ensure that a given society adopts the most appropriate model.

Because the urgency and depth of these issues are relatively new, and such issues usually require some sort of governmental structure to be implemented, we do not have centuries of detailed and nuanced rabbinic guidance for those in search of a Jewish approach to this issue, as compared to other health care–related matters addressed by Jewish law. Instead, guidance from the wisdom of the Jewish tradition on these issues appears in compelling analogous sources in classic Torah literature, which can be extrapolated to the principles and applied to our modern era.[2]

## POTENTIAL PARADIGMS

Contemporary Jewish thinkers have offered many suggestions as to how Judaism might guide us in this dilemma. They point to three main categories within which a diverse—and not necessarily consistent—set of values, directives, and guides may be found:

- *Historical precedent*: Nearly every historically documented Jewish community created some form of a *kupah*, or communal needs fund, which provided medical attention and basic necessities for anyone in the community who could not afford them.[3] Indeed, this model was also a driving force behind the creation of many Jewish hospitals in the United States and elsewhere, as I explore more fully in the next chapter.[4]
- *General Jewish values*: Biblical and rabbinic principles emphasize the following: "Love your neighbor as yourself";[5] *tikkun olam*, or "repairing the world"; the sanctity of life; actualizing holiness, justice, mercy, and the ways of peace; and *pikuach nefesh*, the primacy of life-saving measures, are commonly invoked in discussions about rabbinic perspectives on health care access.[6] The Talmud further mandates that having a resident physician is a basic requirement for any Jewish community.[7] The seminal sixteenth-century Code of Jewish Law, Shulchan Arukh, rules that a doctor who fails to treat a patient is guilty of bloodshed.[8] This is quoted in support of the argument that there is some sort of Jewish communal responsibility to support health care access.[9]
- *Specific Jewish laws*: Jewish law includes a prohibition against standing idly by while another's blood is shed;[10] obligations of charitable giving and the regulation of charity fund distributions;[11] rabbinic rulings related

to forcing ritual circumcizers to perform circumcisions free of charge in cases where a baby's family cannot afford to pay;[12] and the priority of communal responsibilities over the needs of individuals.[13]

Each of these approaches may seem compelling to some but feel forced to others. Either way, none provides a comprehensive paradigm. Moreover, given that so much of Jewish tradition developed when Jews were living in small and somewhat homogenous societies without modern technology or governmental influence (until the founding of the State of Israel), most of these approaches do not fit neatly into contemporary realities and must be combined with various other principles and often reinterpreted widely outside of their original context. Accordingly, I would like to propose an approach to provide systematic guidance on this issue that some others have suggested but has yet to be fully mined for its potential.

## THE SOURCE OF THE COMMANDMENT TO HEAL

Many are under the impression that the verse "You shall surely heal" (*verapo yerapeh*) is the commandment to engage in medical care (Ex. 21:19). However, that verse simply gives physicians permission to engage in a variety of medical activities: to heal even though they might think doing so goes against the divine will, to attempt to heal even illnesses that one might regard as the result of a divinely ordained decree, to engage in medical risk, and to charge for medical services.[14] However, according to many, the verse that commands healing is actually the precept of returning a lost object (Deut. 22:2–3).[15] The great medieval rabbinic thinker Maimonides explains that "this verse includes returning a person's body, for if one sees them dying and can save them, one should save them, whether physically, monetarily, or with knowledge."[16]

## THE SCOPE AND IMPLICATIONS OF THE COMMANDMENT

The laws of returning lost objects go beyond interpersonal relationships. Some commentaries explain that the purpose of these Torah requirements is to facilitate the very foundations of an ethical government/country.[17] In addition to the positive requirement to return lost objects, this verse also includes a prohibition against disregarding others' lost objects, which can be seen as a general prohibition against ignoring the plight of those who are suffering or lacking.[18]

Using the commandment to return a lost object as the paradigm for understanding communal health care responsibilities allows us to reframe the issue. One may be said to have a legitimate expectation to have their lost objects returned, which means we may even be able to speak of a *right* for all to receive health care.[19] Such an expectation is a result of the fact that a community, society, or perhaps a government has an obligation or at the very least there is an ideal to strive to provide access to basic health care requirements for all of its members.[20] Indeed, from a Jewish perspective, the primary emphasis should be less on rights and much more on an analysis of obligations and social responsibilities to ensure the promotion of health and human dignity, as discussed in the introduction to this book.[21]

The laws of returning lost objects have their own system of detailed and nuanced rules, many of which can be applied to our modern context. For example, there are numerous requirements in these laws intended to prevent objects from becoming lost in the first place, such as the ruling that if one sees impending flood waters that may damage or displace another's property, one is obligated to create a protective barrier.[22] Providing access to preventive medicine might be considered a requirement under this rubric because providing medicine to prevent damage to one's body is analogous to constructing a barrier to prevent damage to one's property. On the other hand, not all found objects require returning, such as those of very minimal value, and one is not required to expend excessive effort to locate the owners of a found object or an object itself.[23] Perhaps these boundaries imply that there should be some reasonable limits to universal health care rights. Indeed, there is a sense of partnership in the laws of returning lost objects. For example, one who finds something and knows to whom it belongs may simply return it to the place where the owner is known to be at a certain time each day, but that finder is not obligated to concern themselves with the object any further since the owner will most likely see it.[24]

This approach implies that while the community has an obligation to provide health care, the *individual* is also required to do their part in seeking out health care and conducting themselves in accordance with medical instructions. Furthermore, another limit to health care providers' expectations is implied by the fact that one is not required to return a lost object if doing so will cause damage to others, and thus a health care provider isn't always expected to engage in treating one patient if doing so will inflict harm on another patient.[25]

However, even if a patient is noncompliant, they should not be given up on quickly, especially when matters are out of their control, for the rabbis state that if a person returned someone's animal but it constantly escapes, they are obligated to return it again and again, even if this situation recurs a hundred times.[26] Indeed, the laws of returning lost objects stipulate that even when a person is not expected to return an object, if they began to return an animal but then caused it to wander off even further from its owner's property, they become obligated to return it.[27] This may teach us that if a health care professional is responsible for the deterioration of their patient's condition, they become obligated to help rectify the situation.[28] This could also be very relevant in informing discussions related to patient abandonment. The laws of returning lost objects also maintain that the entire time one is engaged in returning an object, including traveling with the object to its owner, is considered to be part of the mitzvah.[29] This may suggest that since health care professionals are engaged in a mitzvah, perhaps they deserve to be compensated for their travel time in addition to the time they actually spend with patients.[30]

## CONCLUSION

There are many rulings about lost objects, and while several certainly don't fit neatly into public health care policy, there are intriguing possibilities. For example, in addition to the suggestions above, does the ruling that there is no requirement to return objects that were intentionally lost suggest that one who deliberately hurts themselves or jeopardizes their well-being does not have the same rights to communal health care as those who behave more responsibly?[31] Might there be a way to analogize the rulings related to priorities in returning lost objects to triaging health care spending?[32] Might the detailed rules related to returning objects based on their identifying marks (*simanim*) have implications for advance directives, or might the laws of guarding lost objects help inform malpractice theory?

There is much to investigate, but, suffice it to say, this area may be the most relevant analog for determining contemporary communal health care policy and a bioethics of responsibility, and it deserves more attention. Of course, any such policy would need to consider other Jewish values, laws, and principles in addition to modern public health strategies and economics, but there is a need for one overarching Jewish principle to guide this discussion instead of multiple forced attempts.[33] The laws of returning lost objects seem to constitute the best candidate for this endeavor.

# NOTES

1. A. Steinberg, *HaRefuah KeHalakhah*, vol. 1 (Jerusalem: printed by the author, 2017), 5, 107.

2. See similar discussion related to civilian casualties in war in Responsa *Minchat Asher, Devarim*, 218.

3. *Sefer Likutim (Machberet 2)* of Rabbi R. Malki (Rav and doctor in Jerusalem in the mid-fifteenth century), cited in *Tzitz Eliezer* 15:40(7). See also *Mishneh Torah, Hilkhot Matnot Aniyim* 9:1–3. See also discussion of importance of supporting Jewish hospitals and communal health care funds in *Minchat Asher–Magefat HaKorona*, 12. Other phrases for this in Jewish history have included a *hekdesh* room set aside in synagogues for care of sick itinerants since ancient times and *krankenhausen* Jewish homes for the sick throughout Europe. Alan M. Kraut and Deborah A. Kraut, *Covenant of Care: Newark Beth Israel and the Jewish Hospital in America* (New Brunswick, NJ: Rutgers University Press, 2007), 2.

4. See discussion in Kraut and Kraut, *Covenant of Care*, 2–3; and Jill Jacobs, *There Shall Be No Needy: Pursuing Social Justice through Jewish Law and Tradition* (Woodstock, VT: Jewish Lights, 2009), 171–75. Similarly, in late medieval times Jewish communities around the world maintained hospitals, communal physicians, nurses, midwives, and visitation societies, and the sages ruled that communities could divert gifts or legacies given for building synagogues to construction of hospitals or any form of aid to the sick. See Jonathan Sacks, *To Heal a Fractured World: The Ethics of Responsibility* (New York: Schocken, 2005), 48.

5. *Tzitz Eliezer* 15:40(7).

6. See summary in Jeff Levin, "Jewish Ethical Themes That Should Inform the National Healthcare Discussion: A Prolegomenon," *Journal of Religion and Health* 51, no. 3 (2012): 589, https://doi.org/10.1007/s10943-012-9617-6.

7. *Sanhedrin* 17a (the Rambam lists this requirement first in *Hilkhot De'ot* 4:23).

8. *Shulchan Arukh* in YD 336:1.

9. See Rabbi S. Goren, *Torat HaRefuah*, 292–308. In addition to these reasons, Rabbi Zilberstein adds that if it was up to the *beit din*, salaries would certainly be provided for doctors since the *Mishnah Berurah* (306:24) rules that just as a midwife may accept payment for services provided on Shabbat so that she will not be lax in her duties, so too the same must apply to doctors. *Shiurei Torah LeRofim* 1, 200 and 227.

10. Nachum Amsel, *Encyclopedia of Jewish Values between Man and Man* (Jerusalem: Urim, 2018), 393; and Nochum Mangel and Shmuel Klatzin, "What Does the Torah Say about Obamacare?" Chabad.org, n.d., https://www.chabad.org/library/article_cdo/aid/1914545/jewish/What-Does-the-Torah-Say-About-Obamacare.htm.

11. Chaim Apfel, "Government-Mandated Healthcare: Halakha and Social Policy," *Verapo Yerape* 3 (2011): 95–110. Apfel points out that obligations of *tzedakah* require support of those who are lacking basic needs as well as societal obligations to help bring financial stability and strengthen the poor; thus, a government must provide for their poor, and the *Shulchan Arukh* in YD 248:1–2 requires setting up communal funds. See also Michael Broyde, "Healthcare Reform: A Jewish Perspective," Torah Cafe, n.d., https://www.torahcafe.com

/torahcafemobile/video/abo3a9a21; and Aaron L. Mackler, "Judaism, Justice, and Access to Health Care," *Kennedy Institute of Ethics Journal* 1, no. 2 (June 1991): 134.

12. *Tzitz Eliezer* 5, *Ramat Rachel* 24:3–6, citing Rema, YD 261:1 and *Teshuvah MeAhavah*, which says that based on the ruling that a ritual circumcizer must perform circumcisions for free when necessary, a rabbinic court can also force a physician to treat an indigent patient for free, from which it can be inferred that society itself is obligated to fulfill the requirement of circumcision and providing medical care for everyone, including the indigent, and thus, argues the *Tzitz Eliezer*, a rabbinic court should appoint a government agency to do so. See also the discussion in Rabbi J. David Bleich, "Survey of Recent Halakhic Periodical Literature," *Tradition* 21, no. 3 (Fall 1984): 83. A related argument is that Jewish law compares physicians to judges, who are both supposed to be communally licensed and hired, receiving payment from communal funds, not individuals. Therefore, it is argued, there is a Jewish social duty to provide both health care and a court system as a public social service. David Novak, *The Sanctity of Human Life* (Washington, DC: Georgetown University Press, 2007), 102–4.

13. Steinberg, *HaRefuah KeHalakhah*, 5, 108. Professor Steinberg argues that the prohibition against paying a ransom for more than a person is worth—even if an individual wants to pay the ransom, since it could lead to future danger to the community—shows us that there are communal rights that override individual needs. Similarly, the ruling of the Rashba (4:185), that a Jewish community can force every member to pay for whatever they determine is a communal need, implies that if a legitimate government decides that something is a necessity, people can be compelled to pay for it. Amsel, *Encyclopedia of Jewish Values between Man and Man*, 398. Rabbi S. Goren also proves from numerous sources, such as the obligation of local rabbinic courts to ensure functional roads and communal infrastructure, that the responsibility of the health of a community does not fall on individual doctors but is a communal responsibility that must be ensured by rabbinic courts and communal leaders (*Torat HaRefuah*, 313–16). See also Responsa *Aseh Lekha Rav* 7:70.

14. On going against divine will, see Rashi, *Bava Kamma* 85a, s.v. *nitna*. On healing illnesses perhaps resulting from a divinely ordained decree, see *Tosafot, Bava Kamma* 85a, s.v. *shenitna*; *Tosafot Ri HaChasid, Berakhot* 60a, s.v. *mikan*; and *Moshav Zekenim, Shemot* 21:19. On engaging in medical risk and charging for medical services, see Ramban, *Torat HaAdam, Sha'ar HaSakanah*; and Responsa *Da'at Kohen* 140.

15. *Sifrei Devarim* 22:3; and *Bava Kamma* 81b; *Sanhedrin* 73a.

16. Commentary to Mishnah, *Nedarim* 4:4.

17. *Sefer HaChinuch*, Mitzvah 538; and *Ralbag*, Deut. 22, *HaTo'elet HaShevi'i*. Additionally, there is a prohibition against being paid for certain mitzvot, such as teaching Torah, returning lost objects, or providing medical care. *Shulchan Arukh*, YD 336:2. Since one can receive payment for returning lost objects for the time they spent not working (*schar batala*—see *Bava Metzia* 30b and 31b), Rabbi H. Schachter argues that a community is required to have a fund by which to pay doctors a salary, as a type of *schar batala* so they won't get other jobs and thereby be unavailable to practice medicine. *Ginat Egoz*, 185–87.

18. *Mishneh Torah, Gezelah VaAvedah* 11:1. Many commentators see the purpose of these laws as developing kindness and compassion for others (Rabbeinu Bachya, Deut. 22:1; Abarbanel, Deut. 22; and Rambam, *Moreh Nevukhim* 3:40).

19. Although it could be argued that this is also a matter of *obligation*, namely of the finder to return the lost object, perhaps the owner of the item also has a *right* to have it retuned since the finder must safeguard an object whose owner can be identified and is held responsible to pay the owner back if any damage occurs to the item, such that the owner can claim their *right* to their object, or its value, from the finder (*Mishneh Torah, Gezelah VaAvedah* 13:10; and *Shulchan Arukh*, CM 267:16).

20. Perhaps a stronger case can be made from a Jewish perspective for a communal obligation to provide health care than a government obligation to do so because, as Rabbi Jonathan Sacks argues, "The Torah established the first form of what came to be known as a welfare state—with one significant difference. It did not depend on a *state*. It was part of *society*, implemented not by power but by moral responsibility, not by governments but by individuals in local communities." Jonathan Sacks, *Covenant & Conversation, a Weekly Reading of the Jewish Bible: Deuteronomy; Renewal of the Sinai Covenant* (New Milford, CT: Maggid, 2019), 16, 133. Rabbi Sacks's concern is that when government takes responsibility for these social needs, it robs citizens of the opportunity to perform the altruism necessary to maintain a free society. However, since private charity and volunteering is insufficient to correct some of the huge inequities in society, what is needed is to find the proper balance between governmental support and communal relationships. Jonathan Sacks, *The Home We Build Together: Moving beyond Multiculturalism* (London: Continuum, 2007), 128–31.

21. In this chapter we will not enter the debate of the "right" to health care versus the "right" to freedom from coercion or the "rights" of the medical profession.

22. *Bava Metzia* 31a; *Mishneh Torah, Gezelah VaAvedah* 11:20. Similarly, if a cow is found pasturing among vineyards, one is obligated to return the animal to its owner to prevent damage to the property. *Mishneh Torah, Gezelah VaAvedah* 15:4; see also *Shulchan Arukh HaRav, Metzia UPikadon*, 33.

23. *Bava Metzia* 27a; and *Mishneh Torah, Gezelah VaAvedah* 11:12. For example, the Talmud in *Bava Metzia* 28a–b (and codified in *Mishneh Torah, Gezelah VaAvedah* 13:8–10) states that during the times of the Temple a lost object would not need to be announced perpetually, but for each of the next three festivals was sufficient. After the destruction of the Temple, the lost object was announced in the synagogue, and then it was enough to simply ask one's neighbors, and if no one came forward, it would remain with the one who found it (this paradigm deserves further exploration as it could provide the basis of an exploration related to the infrastructure a community would need to establish in order to enable an environment with as few lost objects as possible, which could then be applied to health care). Furthermore, the Talmud rules that one is required to return a lost object that they can see, which is within 1 in 7-1/2 mil (a Talmudic measurement of distance) or about 3,000–4,000 feet, but one would not be required to go out of their way to find a lost object beyond that (*Bava Metzia* 33a). Although this discussion relates to unburdening an animal, *Tosafot HaRosh* says it applies to returning lost objects as well.

24. *Bava Kamma* 57a; and *Mishneh Torah, Gezelah VaAvedah* 11:15.

25. *Shiurei Torah LeRofim* 6:318, 62–63.

26. *Bava Metzia* 31a; and *Mishneh Torah, Gezelah VaAvedah* 11:14.

27. *Bava Batra* 88a.

28. *Shiurei Torah LeRofim* 6:425, 419.

29. *Nimukei Yosef, Bava Metzia* 16a.

30. *Shiurei Torah LeRofim* 6:342, 139.

31. *Shiurei Torah LeRofim* 11:11. For example, the *Minchat Chinuch* (*Kometz HaMinchah*, Mitzvah 237), rules that there is no mitzvah to save someone who attempts to take their own life. Rabbi B. H. Epstein rules similarly in *Tosefet Brachah* on Lev. 19:16. See Benjamin Freedman, *Duty and Healing: Foundations of a Jewish Bioethic* (New York: Routledge, 1999), 150–51. However, many *poskim* disagree because, although one has the right to lose their own property, people do not own their bodies and thus do not have the right to damage themselves (*Teshuvot VeHanhagot* 3:366; *Minchat Asher, Devarim*, 251; and *Shiurei Torah LeRofim* 6:426, 423, and 6:427, 427n3). Indeed, the triage protocols adopted by the Israeli Ministry of Health in May 2020 during the COVID-19 pandemic stated that circumstances that may be considered to be the patient's fault, such as negligence that may have caused a COVID-19 infection, should not be included in making triage decisions. "Position Paper: Triage Decisions for Severely Ill Patients during the COVID-19 Pandemic," Joint Commission for the Israel National Council on Bioethics, the Ethics Bureau of the Israel Medical Association and the Israeli Ministry of Health, May 2020, https://www.health.gov.il/PublicationsFiles/position -paper-230520.pdf. Rabbi Zilberstein suggests that in a triage situation, an argument could be made for prioritizing one who was careful about their health over one who caused their own illness but that since both patients support the health care system by paying taxes, they both deserve equal rights to treatment (*Shiurei Torah LeRofim* 6:426, 423, and 6:427).

32. *Mishneh Torah, Gezelah VaAvedah* 12:1–2.

33. Jonathan Sacks, *Future Tense: Jews, Judaism, and Israel in the Twenty-First Century* (New York: Schocken, 2009), 226.

# CHAPTER FOUR

# Jewish Hospitals in America

In addition to exploring crucial Jewish values, as I have done throughout this book, it is also essential to study history in order to appreciate how core elements of social and personal responsibility have been incorporated into Jewish communal life in response to changing social needs and circumstances.[1] This communal history is both instructive and inspiring. The lessons of the past are especially important since history tends to repeat itself, as the story of Jewish hospitals in America illustrates. This chapter provides a detailed overview of the history of Jewish hospitals in America, followed by my suggestions as to what Jewish hospitals could mean to the Jewish community and our society at large going forward.

Among the first Jews to arrive in North America were a group of twenty-three refugees from Brazil who made their way to New Amsterdam (New York City) in 1654. They were not welcomed warmly, as Peter Stuyvesant, the Dutch director general of the colony, initially tried to block their entry. He relented and permitted them to enter only on the condition that they would pledge to ensure that the poor among them would not become a burden on the community and would agree to take responsibility for supporting them.[2] The Jewish community internalized this expectation and worked hard to avoid stirring public resentment. This "sacred promise" to the larger society to care for their own became known as "the Stuyvesant Pledge."[3] As the American Jewish community slowly grew, they created their own voluntary social support including educational, health, and welfare systems to try not to be a societal burden, similar to what they had previously done in other countries (see chapter 3), which eventually led to founding Jewish hospitals in the mid-nineteenth century.[4]

# FIRST WAVE

Jewish hospitals in the United States were founded in three waves. The first wave began in 1850 as a shortage of hospital beds developed across the United States, primarily as a result of urban epidemics, such as cholera and yellow fever outbreaks.[5] The founders of these first Jewish hospitals expressed feelings of shame when they were unable to take care of their own.[6] They framed their goal not only as an attempt to avoid becoming a burden but primarily as a positive mission of obligation and responsibility to live up to Jewish values of *tzedakah* (charity/righteousness) and *bikur cholim* (visiting the sick).[7] The founders of these hospitals thus spoke with a strong sense of purpose to be of assistance to the sick and the poor.[8]

However, there was also a negative impetus for founding these hospitals. As a minority group, Jews tried not to complain publicly, but another motive became apparent in internal publications and discussions. At that time, anti-Semitism was increasing, and there were also widespread attempts at converting sick Jews in American hospitals, often including forced readings of Christian scriptures as well as deathbed conversions and baptisms.[9] The most desperately ill Jews were the most vulnerable. Jewish hospitals were thus needed for protection and to provide culturally sensitive care, where patients had access to kosher food, a rabbi, and a range of religious services and where no one would ever be turned away due to an inability to pay.[10]

Although there was initially some debate over whether these hospitals should be exclusively for Jews, the consensus quickly became that Jews should not treat others the way they had been treated by excluding others and that perhaps by welcoming all people, they would reduce anti-Semitism and create goodwill for the Jewish community.[11] Furthermore, there was a recognition that Jewish law requires Jews to "sustain the poor who are not Jewish along with poor Jews, and visit the sick who are not Jewish along with sick Jews, and one buries the dead who are not Jewish along with dead Jews, because these are the ways of peace."[12]

From the earliest days of Jewish hospitals in America, Jews were thus very proud that all people in need were equally welcomed by them.[13] For example, at the opening ceremony for the Jewish Hospital in Denver in 1889, it was announced that its goal was to "rear a Temple unbounded by any creed. As pain knows no creed, so is this building the prototype of the grand idea of Judaism, which casts aside no stranger no matter of what race or blood."[14] In New York it was declared that "Beth Israel, like Abraham's tent, will be open to sufferers without distinction as to race or creed."[15] There are numerous examples of this type of inclusive sentiment at Jewish hospitals at that time.[16]

## SECOND WAVE

From the late 1880s until the 1920s, over two million Eastern European Jews immigrated to the United States, and during that period the number of Jewish hospitals in America increased fivefold.[17] These immigrants tended to be poor, religiously observant, and frequently resented by many Americans at the time, thus exacerbating much of the impetus for Jewish hospitals during the first wave.[18] Furthermore, the disproportionately high volume of Jewish tuberculosis patients at this time triggered a nationwide effort to create Jewish hospitals and relief societies to care for Jewish patients.[19]

Despite the Jewish community's effort to care for their own sick, many Jews had to seek care outside their community, where they were again subjected not only to cultural insensitivity but also to severe mistreatment and sometimes even physical assaults.[20] American physicians began labeling Jewish patients as being "subhuman," "dirty," "nervous," and "difficult," and they even created specific phrases and diagnoses for them, such as "Hebraic Debility," and "Jew-Neurasthenia."[21] Needless to say, Jewish patients did not receive proper medical care at most hospitals and needed to be sheltered from the consequences of this type of prejudice. Of course, most Jewish physicians would have the necessary language skills and cultural sensitivity to mitigate some of these concerns, but then another problem developed that exacerbated the need for Jewish hospitals.

Whereas in the nineteenth century most physicians apprenticed with private physicians in home-based practices, in the twentieth century this training transitioned to medical schools and hospitals.[22] However, for the first half of the twentieth century, anti-Semitic policies restricted Jewish medical school graduates' access to internship and residency programs, and Jews were denied staff privileges in hospitals, while the few who had access were subject to harassment and verbal abuse.[23] In the 1920s many American hospitals would not accept any Jews on their medical staff, and if Jewish physicians wanted to find a hospital to accept their patients, they could usually do so only by making a referral via a non-Jewish colleague.[24] If they could get their patients admitted at all, Jewish doctors found that they often had to wait weeks longer than non-Jewish doctors to do so.[25] In some cases a hospital's medical staff even went on strike and made physical threats to prevent Jewish doctors from being hired and to force them to be fired or resign.[26] Jews also faced difficulty in the area of medical school education. For example, in 1927 many medical schools had restricted personnel policies such that of the thousand Jewish physicians in New York City at that time, not one of them held a full-fledged professorship in any medical school that was part of a university.[27]

On top of that, and perhaps most significantly for the history of Jewish hospitals in America, medical schools used many methods of determining whether an applicant was Jewish, in which case they were often denied admission. Quotas were put into place on the number of Jews that medical schools would accept, so, for example, between 1920 and 1940, when these quotas took effect, Jewish enrollment at Columbia's College of Physicians fell from 47 percent to 6 percent.[28] Similarly, Cornell Medical School's percentage of Jewish students dropped from 40 percent to 5 percent during that time.[29] Those Jews who did manage to graduate from medical school at that time were often denied residencies in non-Jewish hospitals and were refused hospital privileges after graduation.[30]

The need for Jewish physicians to have the ability to freely train, practice medicine, and care for their patients in hospitals became the primary impetus for the development of many of the Jewish clinics and hospitals between 1912 and 1936.[31] These hospitals faced many obstacles as they often had a hard time finding anyone to sell them land for a Jewish hospital, and national accrediting boards frequently didn't approve or allow graduate residencies at Jewish hospitals, even though these institutions met the accreditation standards.[32] Despite these challenges, the Jewish community rallied around this cause as communal Jewish federations allocated approximately 25 percent of their local grants to Jewish hospitals.[33] Jewish hospitals were often the Jewish community's most impressive and identifiable philanthropy in each city, and because even Jewish philanthropy was not accepted by the broader society at this time, Jewish hospitals were one of the few ways that individual Jews could give to humanity.[34]

## THIRD WAVE AND BEYOND

There was also a brief third wave of development of Jewish hospitals during the 1940s and 1950s, spurred by the Hospital Survey and Construction Act of 1946 (also known as the Hill–Burton Act), which created thousands of new hospital beds, primarily in suburban areas.[35] This legislation had a significant impact on the older Jewish hospitals, which were mostly located in urban areas, enabling many of them to relocate, merge, or create new hospitals. Quotas limiting Jews came to an end in the 1960s thanks to a combination of societal attitudes and government policies, but these hospitals remained welcoming places for Jews to seek care and employment, and they made sure to publicize the fact that patients and staff of all backgrounds remained equally welcomed in them.[36] Even as demographics changed and many historically Jewish hospitals were gradually made up primarily of people who were not Jewish, these institutions continued to articulate the same sense of purpose to care for all people who were suffering in their communities.[37]

The need for Jewish hospitals gradually declined. Jews were allowed to seek care and employment at any hospital, and many non-Jewish hospitals even opened kosher kitchens or created access to Jewish religious needs.[38] The Medicare and Medicaid plans that were developed in the 1960s made hospitals less dependent on private philanthropy, and by 1981 Jewish federations allocated only 2.3 percent of their funding to health care and hospitals (a number that has continued to shrink since then[39]).[40] Furthermore, the attitude toward anti-Semitism gradually shifted from combating it via philanthropy to fighting it head-on through organizations such as the Anti-Defamation League.[41] The hospital industry also became much more competitive at this time, and financial pressures forced many smaller community hospitals to merge with larger systems or close.[42]

Throughout American history there have been 113 Jewish hospitals in twenty-four American cities, but twenty-four of them had merged with other Jewish hospitals, thirty-five had closed, and twenty-four had been purchased by or merged with non-Jewish hospitals by 2012, leaving just twenty-two remaining independent.[43] As of 2022 estimates are that there are only about ten left, and possibly as few as five, depending on how one defines a Jewish hospital.[44]

## WHAT HAS IT MEANT TO BE A JEWISH HOSPITAL?

Christian hospitals in America are typically built on a strong church base, with articles of incorporation that guarantee the sponsoring church or organization will maintain a formal role in its governance, and often including precise ethical and religious directives of operation.[45] Jewish hospitals in America, on the other hand, have no such structure or official association. How exactly to define what it has meant to be a "Jewish hospital" has been the subject of much debate, and the difference between a Jewish hospital and a hospital for Jews is not always clear. At earlier periods in American history, some suggested that for a hospital to be considered a Jewish hospital, some of the following attributes must apply:[46]

- It was founded primarily by members of the Jewish community.
- It was built primarily for members of the Jewish community.
- It was funded primarily by members of the Jewish community.
- It has a Jewish name.
- It is governed primarily by members of the Jewish community.

- It is staffed by an especially high percentage of Jews.
- It is viewed as "Jewish" by the Jewish community.
- It adheres to Jewish religious or ritual practice to a greater degree than other religions or ritual practices.
- It is a place in which Jewish patients feel comfortable (likely including cultural sensitivity, not displaying symbols from other faith traditions, and in-language care).

## WHAT DOES IT MEAN TO BE A JEWISH HOSPITAL IN AMERICA TODAY?

The obvious question that arises is whether there is still a need for Jewish hospitals in America today. There is a certain integrity or sacred trust to the founders of these hospitals to maintain the institutions that they founded and built, but are they still needed for any uniquely Jewish reasons? Anti-Semitism is still a concern in the Jewish community, and it remains important to promote goodwill and maintain an infrastructure in case of a severe resurgence of anti-Semitism in society or within the medical establishment.[47] People often also praise the sense of community, comradery, and tradition at Jewish hospitals. But I believe that what makes them unique is far deeper. I suggest that the survival of some proudly Jewish hospitals in America today is crucial to maintaining essential areas of focus in the tapestry of our health care system. The rich and impressive history of Jewish hospitals in America serves as a powerful reminder and incentive for these hospitals to maintain fidelity to certain profound ideals, which will hopefully serve as role models for others.

### Inclusivity

Jewish hospitals, by their very existence and hopefully by their example, teach the importance of inclusivity and welcoming the stranger. The Hebrew Bible uses the story of the Jewish people's slavery in Egypt as national moral education intended to transform their perspective of humanity and morality.[48] Right after the exodus narrative, the Torah gives numerous commands to remind the people to learn these lessons not just as knowledge but as shared memory of their own experience.[49] The Torah, in multiple places, is therefore very clear about the obligation to love the stranger.[50] For example, it commands, "Do not wrong or oppress the stranger for you yourselves were once strangers in the land of Egypt" (Ex. 22:21) and "Do not oppress the stranger, for you know what it feels like to be a stranger, for you yourselves were once strangers in the land of Egypt" (Ex. 23:9).[51]

So, too, remembering the difficult history that led to the creation of Jewish hospitals in America should continue to sensitize and inspire contemporary Jewish hospitals to embody these crucial lessons. Having lived and suffered as strangers at many points of Jewish history, Jews are obligated by the Torah to become people who are especially dedicated to caring for strangers.[52] Jewish hospitals were necessary in America because they were a place for people who otherwise were excluded, alienated, isolated, or unwelcome in the broader society to feel safe and at home. Remembering what it was like for Jews to be victims, a Jewish hospital must therefore be a place where all people feel comfortable and welcome, not with the intention of encouraging them to become Jewish but simply as an act of solidarity and identification with the stranger.

It is therefore no coincidence that in 1906 the Jewish Kaspare Cohn Hospital in Los Angeles hired the first female physician to practice in Los Angeles, Sarah Vasen, who went on to become the hospital's superintendent. That hospital later changed its name to Cedars of Lebanon and, along with many other American Jewish hospitals, became a safe haven for Jewish physicians who were driven out of Germany during the Nazi era.[53] Another important example of the enduring values of Jewish hospitals relates to their involvement in the civil rights movement. For example, in 1947 the Jewish Hospital of Cincinnati hired two African American physicians in opposition to Jim Crow laws, and in 1951, Louisville Jewish Hospital hired Jesse Bell, the first African American doctor to practice at a non–African American hospital in that region.[54]

This is an example of particularity leading to universalism. Ironically, in this case, if fidelity to a people's own history and identity is maintained, they can be motivated to be more inclusive and welcoming to others. It is less of a challenge to love one's neighbor who is part of the same community than it is to love the stranger, who some people might regard with fear or animosity.[55] Jewish hospitals are a profound reminder that not only is "love your neighbor as yourself" a foundation of Jewish medical ethics but so is the crucial commitment to "love the stranger." Remembering this history places a special obligation on Jewish hospitals to embrace marginalized populations.

## Faith-Friendly, Not Faith Enforced

Jewish hospitals serve as unique models of faith-based institutions because, unlike those under the auspices of some other faiths, Jewish hospitals do not impose any specific religious directives of practice. A Jewish hospital should indeed be a place that is faith-friendly and a place where religious practice is facilitated but not a place where it is enforced. A lesson that Jewish communities have learned over the course of their history is that not only have Jews frequently had other religions imposed on them (as mentioned earlier), and not only is religious coercion usually ineffective at promoting religion and risks anti-religious backlash, but, perhaps counterintuitively, it is bad for religion.[56] As Rabbi Jonathan Sacks taught, religion truly acquires influence only when it relinquishes power and instead becomes the voice of the voiceless and the conscience of the community.[57] Religion can thrive without exerting power, and many rabbinic thinkers posit that religious acts truly have value only when they are done free of any coercion.[58] Religion is at its best, Rabbi Sacks taught, when it relies on the strength of example and at its worst when it seeks to impose truth by force.[59] The phrase "religious coercion" is thus an oxymoron. One cannot impose truth or spirituality by force;[60] as the Talmud rules, "Coerced agreement is not consent."[61]

This is why some leading rabbinic thinkers have argued that according to Jewish law governments should always limit their authority to the civil realm and never involve themselves in religious matters.[62] Indeed, some suggest that it was the American separation of church and state that created the reality that religion has no power but enormous influence, and this can be true for Jewish hospitals as well.[63]

At the same time, however, steps are often taken in Jewish hospitals to ensure that religion can indeed be fully practiced by those who *choose* to do so. One example is the development of "reasonable accommodation" policies to facilitate religious patients' abilities to receive treatment in accordance with their own values and to provide a practical and compassionate way to resolve conflicts.[64] Such policies are important ways in which the faith-based practices or beliefs of religious patients can be enabled without being forced on all patients in a given institution. While such accommodations are beneficial to many populations, they may prove to be especially important to the rapidly growing Orthodox Jewish community and could revive a very relevant need for Jewish hospitals where they can obtain religiously/culturally congruent care.[65]

The fact that Jewish hospitals accommodate religious needs but don't dictate them can also be helpful when it comes to procedures that other faith-based hospitals prohibit, such as abortions, but that Judaism sometimes allows and in certain situations may even require. Since all legal, standard-of-practice procedures are permitted at Jewish hospitals, one who wants to fully observe one's religion is able to do so if one chooses to, which is often not the case when one religious tradition dictates the range of permitted medical practices for all of its staff and patients.

## Values

Examining the history and mission of Jewish hospitals in America also reminds us that there remain certain values that are widely recognized but always in need of encouragement and deeper focus:[66]

- *Research and education*: Jewish hospitals' roots in providing institutions where Jewish medical students can train is a reminder of the centrality of education and rigorous research in Judaism.[67] Early in their history, American Jewish hospitals developed a reputation for innovation, thanks in part to the emphasis on education in the Jewish community.[68] At a time when many faith-based institutions place limits on the types of research they permit, such as some forms of stem-cell research, Jewish hospitals ensure robust access to potentially lifesaving innovation. Education is a core Jewish value that ensures high-quality medicine, promotes human dignity and resilience in challenging times, and is thus central to the practice of modern medicine.[69]
- *Care for body and soul*: American Jewish hospitals have tended to place great importance on certain inconspicuous but meaningful symbols such as mezuzahs.[70] These powerful religious and cultural symbols in places of science and medicine can serve as reminders that a hospital is not just a place where physical ailments are treated but also a source of holistic care, which goes much deeper. As the traditional Jewish prayer for healing, the *mi sheberach*, declares, we pray for both "a healing of the soul and a healing of the body." Traditional symbols and respect for faith can help humanize and give deeper meaning to health care.
- *Responsibility to care for the sick and the poor*: The history of striving not to be a burden but rather focusing on the duty to care for the sick and poor of one's community is a reminder that health care is about taking on responsibility. Throughout history, Jewish communities have cared for those in need instead of relying on others to do it for them. Jewish hospitals remind us to continue this vital tradition.

Of course, these values sometimes come into conflict with each other and aren't always simple to apply. A difficult but very practical example of implementing the history and mission of being a Jewish hospital arose during the COVID-19 pandemic. As vaccination mandates have been enacted, the only exemptions allowed have been for either medical or religious accommodations. Each institution has taken a different approach about strictness in allowing religious accommodations. For a Jewish hospital this issue presents a significant dilemma because, on the one hand, inclusivity and embracing every individual's right to freely practice their own religion are core aspects of a Jewish hospital's identity and mission. On the other hand, however, care for the vulnerable, the sophisticated practice of the art of healing, and an engagement in the science of research and advanced medicine are also central tenets. This issue therefore requires attempting to sensitively balance the desire to respect everyone's ability to live in accordance with their own sincerely held beliefs with promoting the protection that vaccination offers as well as the communal responsibility and accountability that vaccination engenders. That said, one side often must be chosen, and I believe that, for a Jewish hospital, the duty to protect vulnerable patients outweighs the need to accommodate every single sincerely held belief.

## CONCLUSION

Many of the values discussed in this chapter are not exclusively Jewish, and several of them can be found to some extent at other hospitals today. Many religions and, indeed, those with no religion strive for many similar ideals and commitments. This history may have implications for other faith-based hospitals and perhaps even the entire health care system. My contention is simply that using some teachings of the Jewish tradition and studying its rich recent history can provide a focused sense of purpose and serve as an anchor and inspiration to help clarify many of these values and ensure that they are substantial and firmly rooted. Without this foundation and historical context, it would be less certain that these values become embodied with the same sense of urgency and dedication and transmitted to the next generation. It is therefore essential to remember the past so that we can build a better world.

## NOTES

1. On the importance of studying history in the field of bioethics, see Robert Baker, "How Should Students Learn about Contemporary Implications of Health Professionals' Roles in the Holocaust?" *AMA Journal of Ethics* 23, no. 1 (2021): 31–36.

2. Edward C. Halperin, "The Rise and Fall of the American Jewish Hospital," *Academic Medicine* 87, no. 5 (May 2012): 611.

3. Robert Katz, "Paging Dr. Shylock! Jewish Hospitals and the Prudent Reinvestment of Jewish Philanthropy," in *Religious Giving: For the Love of God*, ed. David Smith (Bloomington: Indiana University Press, 2010), 165.

4. Jonathan D. Sarna, *American Judaism: A History* (New Haven, CT: Yale University Press, 2004), 222.

5. Daniel Ethan Bridge, *The Rise and Development of the Jewish Hospital in America, 1850–1984* (Rabbinical thesis, Hebrew Union College, 1985), 25, 18; and Alan M. Kraut and Deborah A. Kraut, *Covenant of Care: Newark Beth Israel and the Jewish Hospital in America* (New Brunswick, NJ: Rutgers University Press, 2007), 3–4.

6. Bridge, *Rise and Development*, 2.

7. Bridge, 22–24; and Laurie Levin, *Cedars-Sinai: The One-Hundred Year History of Cedars-Sinai Medical Center* (Los Angeles: Cedars-Sinai Medical Center, 2002), introduction.

8. Kraut and Kraut, *Covenant of Care*, 24.

9. Katz, "Paging Dr. Shylock!" 166. For example, during the Civil War, all areas under control of Ulysses S. Grant expelled all Jewish residents from their homes in 1862. Kraut and Kraut, *Covenant of Care*, 3; and Bridge, *Rise and Development*, 25–28. Another good example is from the laying of the cornerstone ceremony in 1866 for Baltimore's Asylum for Israelites. Dr. J. Cohen stated, "Many of us know the instances in which poor co-religionists, stricken down upon the bed of illness in the hands of strangers, have been greatly annoyed and their last moments embittered by the obtrusion of sentiments, in the vain attempt to draw them away from the God of their fathers. It was the occurrence of a case of this kind which a few years ago warmed us up to the necessity of making provisions to protect ourselves." Bridge, *Rise and Development*, 26.

10. Halperin, "Rise and Fall," 611. Additional essential religious services included *mezuzot*, avoidance of autopsies unless it would save a life, a separate room for *brit milah*, availability of a rabbi, services on the various holidays, and in some cases daily prayers and kosher food. See also Bridge, *Rise and Development*, 32, 57, 59, 61. Interestingly, some Jewish hospitals, such as Mount Sinai in New York, had a synagogue before they had an operating room, which shows their priorities at the time. Arthur H. Aufses Jr. and Barbara Niss, *This House of Noble Deeds: The Mount Sinai Hospital, 1852–2002* (New York: New York University Press, 2002), 4. Similar issues arose in Europe around the same time, and these services were so important to many Jews, and the ill treatment they received at non-Jewish hospitals was so bad, that some European Jews reported preferring to be poorly cared for in a Jewish hospital over going to well-established municipal hospitals. Jack Y. Vanderhoek, "A Tale of Two Nineteenth-Century Dutch Jewish Hospitals," *Rambam Maimonides Medical Journal* 11, no. 4 (2020): 6; see also Levin, *Cedars-Sinai*, 14.

11. Levin, 4; and Kraut and Kraut, *Covenant of Care*, 24. Some rabbis opposed opening Jewish hospitals, and there were frequent debates—many of which stalled the opening of these hospitals—about religious perspective, ritual practice, location, and whether the hospital should be "sectarian" (only for Jews) or "nonsectarian" (open for all). See also Bridge, *Rise and Development*, 64; and Katz, "Paging Dr. Shylock!" 166–67.

12. *Gittin* 61a.

13. Bridge, *Rise and Development*, 37, 65. Many Jewish hospitals boasted of having equal numbers of Jewish and non-Jewish patients; see also Levin, *Cedars-Sinai*, 58.

14. Bridge, *Rise and Development*, 38.

15. Kraut and Kraut, *Covenant of Care*, 27.

16. For example, at the dedication in 1908 for a new facility for Newark's Beth Israel, the

community rabbi proclaimed that "while this hospital shall be mainly supported by Jews, it will open its doors just as wide as they can swing to receive the non-Jew who may desire to enter and his religious sentiments shall be carefully safeguarded." Kraut and Kraut, *Covenant of Care*, 33. Similarly, in 1866, Philadelphia's Jewish community opened a nonsectarian hospital that proclaimed right on its entrance, "The Hospital was erected by the voluntary contributions of the Israelites of Philadelphia, and is dedicated to the relief of the sick and wounded without regard to creed, color or nationality." Katz, "Paging Dr. Shylock!" 167.

17. Kraut and Kraut, *Covenant of Care*, 64–66. Just from 1919 to 1922, the number of Jewish hospitals more than doubled.

18. Bridge, *Rise and Development*, 20, 35–37, 57; and Kraut and Kraut, *Covenant of Care*, 4, 21.

19. Bridge, *Rise and Development*, 23.

20. Edward C. Halperin, "'This is a Christian Institution and We Will Tolerate No Jews Here': The Brooklyn Medical Interns Hazings," *American Journal of Medical Sciences* 356, no. 6 (2018): 505–17.

21. Kraut and Kraut, *Covenant of Care*, 5; and Katz, "Paging Dr. Shylock!" 170.

22. Bridge, *Rise and Development*, 29.

23. Halperin, "Rise and Fall," 611.

24. Kraut and Kraut, *Covenant of Care*, 120.

25. Kraut and Kraut, 117.

26. Edward C. Halperin, "'We Do Not Want Him Because He Is a Jew': The Montreal Interns' Strike of 1934," *Annals of Internal Medicine* 174 (2021): 852–57.

27. Kraut and Kraut, *Covenant of Care*, 119.

28. Kraut and Kraut, 118.

29. Kraut and Kraut, 118.

30. Kraut and Kraut, 117.

31. Bridge, *Rise and Development*, 30–31; and Kraut and Kraut, *Covenant of Care*, 24, 117.

32. Kraut and Kraut, *Covenant of Care*, 72, 124–25.

33. Katz, "Paging Dr. Shylock!" 172.

34. Katz, 162; and interview with Jonathan Schreiber, vice president of community engagement at Cedars-Sinai, January 2021.

35. Kraut and Kraut, *Covenant of Care*, 140–41; and Halperin, "Rise and Fall," 611.

36. Edward C. Halperin, "Why Did the United States Medical School Admissions Quota for Jews End?" *American Journal of Medical Sciences* 358, no. 5 (2019): 317–25; and Kraut and Kraut, *Covenant of Care*, 174.

37. Kraut and Kraut, 187.

38. Halperin, "Rise and Fall," 612. Ironically, the reduction of anti-Semitism in the medical profession adversely affected some Jewish hospitals as Jewish doctors and researchers gained more options. Aufses and Niss, *This House of Noble Deeds*, 13. See also Katz, "Paging Dr. Shylock!" 172.

39. Interview with Jonathan Schreiber, vice president of community engagement at Cedars-Sinai, January 2021.

40. Katz, "Paging Dr. Shylock!" 173.

41. Katz, 173.

42. Halperin, "Rise and Fall," 612.

43. Halperin, 612.

44. Halperin, 612; and personal correspondence with Dr. Halperin in January 2021. A current list of American Jewish hospitals can be found at this link (although many of these hospitals no longer identify as being Jewish): https://www.kosherdelight.com/Hospital sUSA.shtml. As of 2016, 18.5 percent of hospitals in the United States were religiously affiliated. Between 2001 and 2016 the number of nonprofit religious hospitals decreased by 38.3 percent, but during this time the number of acute care hospitals that were Catholic owned or affiliated grew by 22 percent, even though the overall number of acute care hospitals decreased by 6 percent. Maryam Guiahi, Patricia E. Helbin, Stephanie B. Teal, Debra Stulberg, and Jeanelle Sheeder, "Patient Views on Religious Institutional Health Care," *Journal of the American Medical Association* 2, no. 12 (2019).

45. Bridge, *Rise and Development*, 9, 52–53, 175; and Halperin, "Rise and Fall," 612.

46. Bridge, *Rise and Development*, 2, 51–52.

47. Katz, "Paging Dr. Shylock!" 176.

48. Jonathan Sacks, *Not in God's Name: Confronting Religious Violence* (New York: Schocken, 2015), 183–84.

49. Sacks, 183–84.

50. Depending on how one counts the commandments, the Torah warns against wronging a stranger either thirty-six or forty-six times, more than any other commandment (*Bava Metzia* 59b).

51. See also Leviticus 19:34.

52. Sacks, *Not in God's Name*, 188. Rabbi Sacks goes so far as to argue that "Judaism is the voice of the other throughout history. The whole of Judaism is about making space for the other." Jonathan Sacks, *Future Tense: Jews, Judaism, and Israel in the Twenty-First Century* (New York: Schocken, 2009), 83.

53. Levin, *Cedars-Sinai*, 63. This was especially crucial given that throughout the United States at that time barriers were created to prevent these Jewish refugee physicians from practicing at other hospitals. Laurel Leff and Robert E. Schoen, "Fighting Prejudice and Absorbing Refugees from Nazism: The National Committee for the Resettlement of Foreign Physicians, 1939–1945," *Annals of Internal Medicine* 174, no. 5 (2021): 680.

54. On the Jewish Hospital of Cincinnati, see E. M. Bluestone, "Study of the Health and Medical Activities of the Federation Agencies in Cincinnati, Ohio," December 28, 1947, 26, 131, American Jewish Archives, Cincinnati, Ohio; on the Louisville Jewish Hospital, see Carol Ely, "Interview with Morris Weiss, August 1, 2016," Jewish Kentucky Oral History Project, accession no. 2016oh252_jk028, https://kentuckyoralhistory.org/ark:/16417 /xt7crj48sc8k; and Hannah Thompson, "Louisville Jewish Hospital's 'Tikkun Olam': A Case Example of Continuity for American Jewish Hospitals" (2019), Dean's Award for Excellence in Undergraduate Scholarship, University of Kentucky, https://uknowledge .uky.edu/cgi/viewcontent.cgi?article=1002&context=libraries_undergraduate_scholarship.

55. Sacks, *Not in God's Name*, 181.

56. Rabbi Joseph Ber Soloveitchik, *Community, Covenant, and Commitment: Selected Letters and Communications of Rabbi Joseph B. Soloveitchik* (Jersey City, NJ: Ktav, 2005), 211. See also Rami Schwartz, "The Political Theology of Rabbi Nachum Eliezer Rabinovitch," *Torah u-Madda Journal* 18 (July 5, 2021): 19. In Rabbi Sacks's words, "When religion seeks power, the result is disastrous, if not immediately then ultimately. The result is tragic for the people, catastrophic for the state, and disastrous for religion. When religion, any religion, seizes power, it forfeits the respect of ordinary, decent righteous people, who once respected it and now fear and resent it. The result is the defeat of religion, the birth of a new secularism, and a desecration of the holy." Jonathan Sacks, *The Home We Build Together: Moving beyond Multiculturalism* (London: Continuum, 2007), 223.

57. Sacks, *Not in God's Name*, 222.

58. Sacks, 236; and Schwartz, "The Political Theology of Rabbi Nachum Eliezer Rabinovitch," 10–11. R. Rabinovitch bases his argument primarily on Maimonides's *Guide to the Perplexed*.

59. Sacks, *Not in God's Name*, 234. See also extensive discussion in Aviezer Ravitzky, "Is a Halakhic State Possible? The Paradox of Jewish Theocracy," *Israel Affairs* 11, no. 1 (2005): 137–64.

60. Sacks, *Not In God's Name*, 225. Rabbi Sacks expands elsewhere that "faith, coerced, is not faith. Worship, forced, is not true worship." Jonathan Sacks, *Covenant & Conversation, a Weekly Reading of the Jewish Bible: Exodus* (New Milford, CT: Maggid, 2010), 197. Rabbi Sacks elaborates on this topic elsewhere, citing numerous rabbinic sources, arguing that (1) although there is an obligation to reprove wrongdoing, it does not apply when it is certain that reproof will not be heeded; (2) today rabbinic authorities rule that coercive punishments would be seen as unwarranted and would therefore not improve but worsen the religious environment and that reduction of the power of coercion prepares the world for the Heavenly Kingdom as society gradually moves toward uncoerced acceptance of Jewish law; and (3) education is Judaism's classic alternative to coercion and is the best way to internalize religion. Jonathan Sacks, *One People? Tradition, Modernity, and Jewish Unity* (Oxford: Littman Library of Jewish Civilization in association with Liverpool University Press, 1993), 218–19.

61. *Shabbat* 88a and *Avodah Zarah* 2b, cited by Sacks in *Not in God's Name* (230) and *Home We Build Together* (198). Rabbi Sacks brings further support for this contention from the fact that the tabernacle was built by voluntary donations "from each whose heart prompts them to give," and it united the nation, whereas Solomon's son Rehoboam caused a civil war and split the nation in two by forcing more labor and taxes on the people against their will. Sacks, *Home We Build Together*, 138–42. Rabbi Sacks also mentions a more pragmatic reason to oppose enshrining religious coercion in law, which is simply that the faith imposing itself on others at one time may eventually no longer be in power and would then face danger of being disadvantaged or even persecuted by another faith at that time (198).

62. Schwartz, "Political Theology of Rabbi Nachum Eliezer Rabinovitch," 12, 17, 24–25.

63. Jonathan Sacks, *Morality: Restoring the Common Good in Divided Times* (New York: Basic, 2020), 254–55.

64. L. Syd M. Johnson, "The Case for Reasonable Accommodation of Conscientious Objections to Declarations of Brain Death," *Journal of Bioethical Inquiry* 13, no. 1 (2016): 105–15;

and Ezra Gabbay and Joseph J. Fins, "Go in Peace: Brain Death, Reasonable Accommodation and Jewish Mourning Rituals," *Journal of Religion and Health* 58 (2019): 1672–86.

65. Ari Feldman and Laura E. Adkins, "Orthodox to Dominate American Jewry in Coming Decades as Population Booms," Forward, June 12, 2018, https://forward.com/news/402663/orthodox-will-dominate-american-jewry-in-coming-decades-as-population/.

66. Feldman and Adkins; and Halperin, "Rise and Fall," 613.

67. See discussion in Katz, "Paging Dr. Shylock!" 175.

68. Kraut and Kraut, *Covenant of Care*, 54.

69. Sacks, *Covenant & Conversation: Exodus*, 79, 138; Jonathan Sacks, *Covenant & Conversation, a Weekly Reading of the Jewish Bible: Numbers* (New Milford, CT: Maggid, 2017), 374; and Jonathan Sacks, *Ceremony & Celebration: Introduction to the Holidays* (New Milford, CT: Maggid, 2017), 280. Rabbi Sacks argues, based on *Bava Batra* 21a, that Jews developed the world's first system of public, universal compulsory education over two thousand years ago because Judaism regards studying as the highest religious value.

70. Halperin, "Rise and Fall," 611.

# CHAPTER FIVE

# Brain Death and Conflict Mitigation

Having explored issues of Jewish hospitals, anti-Semitism, and inclusivity brings us now to a discussion of navigating complex scenarios that sometimes pit health care providers and their patients against each other. Religious or cultural values sometimes conflict with medical standards of practice or law. These distressing conflicts frequently occur at the end of life when stress and tensions are high. When patients and their families do not see eye to eye with their health care provider, instead of working toward collaborative, shared decision-making, there are unfortunately times when health care providers might feel that it is best to override the patient's requests, simply inform them of what they see as the medically appropriate thing to do, and then proceed regardless of what the patient or their family wants.[1] In some cases, clinicians may unilaterally withdraw or withhold life support that they consider inappropriate without seeking permission from the patient or surrogate decision-makers.[2]

To illustrate some of the complexities that might arise and suggest more productive ways of handing different perspectives, I will share a brief hypothetical case study and several suggestions it gives rise to using the example of an important issue that some Orthodox Jews occasionally encounter in the health care system: brain death. This can serve as a helpful example because, despite being a legal definition of death, there are some religions that do not accept this determination, and it has been subjected to increasing challenges and resistance in recent years.[3] Nevertheless, once death is determined by neurological criteria (brain death), hospitals have no legal obligation to artificially maintain the body or provide any medical interventions or treatment, and physiological support is thus usually discontinued.[4] These disputes can lead to terrible strife and conflict, often garnering media attention, and increasingly escalate to the courts.[5] There must be a better way.

## CASE

NK is a thirty-two-year-old man who lost consciousness after having a severe headache. His wife, SK, called an ambulance. NK was intubated in the field by emergency medical technicians and brought to the hospital. When NK was admitted, a cranial computed tomography (CT) scan showed subarachnoid hemorrhage (bleeding in the space that surrounds the brain) and severe hydrocephalus (buildup of fluid in the cavities within the brain) with intraventricular hemorrhage (bleeding into the fluid-filled areas of the brain). Twenty-four hours later, NK remained comatose with no brain stem reflexes.

Dr. T explained to SK that NK was probably "brain dead." SK responded, "We are Orthodox Jews, so we do not believe that death happens until the heart stops." Dr. T explained that the next step would be to determine whether NK has any brain activity. SK agreed to allow Dr. T to examine her husband and clarified, "Regardless of what you find, my husband is alive until his heart stops, so we will continue to keep him on the machines until then."

Dr. T wondered how to respond.

## COMMENTARY

As the rabbi of a large medical center with a significant Orthodox Jewish population, I have frequently supported both Orthodox families and our medical staff in an attempt to sensitively navigate a brain death declaration, which isn't accepted as the definition of death by many Orthodox Jews.[6] Although each situation is unique and must be handled on a case-by-case basis by listening, engaging religious leadership, supporting hospital staff, and practicing cultural humility, clinicians can often identify a care plan for patients who are brain dead that is sensitive to both medical standards of practice and personal religious and cultural values.

## MITIGATING CONFLICT IN BRAIN DEATH

*Listen first:* Regarding the case under discussion, I would encourage the physician to begin by listening carefully to family members, expressing empathy and

respect for their outlook, and affirming that their perspective is important and
that team members will try their best to accommodate it insofar as possible.
The hospital's reasonable accommodation policy should be reviewed (if it has
one; if not, one should be developed).[7] The first goal must be to establish
trust and a positive working relationship. Orthodox or not, everyone needs
time to process such a shock. Furthermore, being treated with compassion by
their health care providers can be beneficial for people who find themselves in
situations like the one in this case.[8] Once the brain death testing as well as con-
firmatory testing (which is often required by Jewish law[9]) is completed, more
time will have passed—which hopefully will help the family to become more
amenable to discussion—and the results of the testing might be relevant for
helping the family and their rabbi determine next steps.

*Involve religious leadership*: If all testing confirms the brain death diagnosis, and
if the family members remain adamant that they do not accept this as the definition of death and thus request ongoing mechanical support, then the next
phase of care for the family begins. The family should continue to be listened to
and shown compassion. Their rabbi as well as supportive professionals within
the hospital, such as a chaplain who is familiar with the religious needs of the
Orthodox community, should be included in discussions.

It is crucial for medical practitioners to establish a collaborative, trusting
relationship with the family's rabbinic leadership. Within Orthodoxy, rabbinic
leadership often plays a strong role in decision-making due to the central
role that Jewish law plays in all decision-making (not just medical decision-
making). The hospital's chaplaincy department often has a good relationship
with local rabbinic leadership and can thus serve as an important liaison by
helping to explain rabbinic rulings to the hospital staff and, conversely, the
medical culture to the rabbinic leadership.

*Support hospital staff*: Some hospital staff members might become distressed by
the prospect of continuing interventions for a body that they consider to be a
corpse. They should receive emotional support, and some should be excused
from caring for the patient if they are not comfortable doing so. In addition
to being the right thing to do and preventing burnout, supporting staff can
help mitigate potential escalation of conflict between frustrated health care
providers and families.

*Practice cultural humility*: For those remaining on the care team, it becomes
essential to reiterate the importance of cultural humility and the fact that de-
fining life and death are philosophical concepts, not just medical criteria. Family members might not see the status of the patient in the same way that the
medical team does, so insisting that they frame everything within the standard
medical worldview will not only come across as disrespectful but also make

effective communication impossible. A different worldview should not automatically render someone "difficult" or maladaptive. It is crucial to remember that family members might still be shocked or experiencing severe anticipatory grief and might turn to their community and religion—as they do for all major decisions—as a source of guidance and support.

Demonstrating true respect for diverse cultures and traditions is especially important in health care, where clear communication and trust is crucial, and it can require a significant amount of effort and dedication on the part of all care providers. Clearly, no one can be an expert in every nuance of faith or ritual for the many ethnic and religious groups that one may encounter in a hospital. That is why instead of striving for "cultural competency," it is suggested that we seek to develop "cultural humility."[10] Cultural humility, the way I am suggesting the concept, recognizes that everyone is different, so instead of assuming that one can know everything they need to know about a given culture or community, one should be inquisitive, curious, and open to learning about each individual that they encounter and should strive to care for every patient in accordance with that person's own unique values and lived experience.

*Coming to a compromise*: A reasonable amount of time should be allowed to reach a compromise, and like all clinical judgments, "reasonable" is based on the particulars of each situation but is usually a few days (in my experience, brain-dead patients' hearts often stop on their own after a few days, although this sometimes takes longer, especially in younger patients). At the same time, the family should be shown compassion, understanding, and emotional support. If there is still no clinical change, institutional pressure to remove life-sustaining technologies might begin to build, as will stress and anxiety. At this phase we usually attempt to figure out a compromise approach as we move toward a resolution.

While decisions are made on a case-by-case basis, taking various crucial details into account, most rabbinic leaders are reasonable and can help find a workable approach. For example, while those who interpret Jewish law as not accepting neurological criteria for determining death will generally not permit active withdrawal of life support, they do often permit withholding increased interventions. This exception is based partially on the distinction that Jewish law makes between "withholding" and "withdrawing." Jewish law sometimes permits withholding life-prolonging interventions in dying patients since it is passive.[11] However, Jewish law considers stopping therapy to be the performance of an action. Thus, while terminal extubation will rarely be permitted, there are times when rabbis will permit not adding any new medical interventions, not increasing vent settings in the face of pulmonary decline, or not engaging in chest compressions when the heart stops. Sometimes they will also allow some medications, for example, vasopressors, to run out and not be refilled. This approach, which can be very helpful, is sometimes referred to as Do Not Escalate (DNE). DNE recognizes the desire not to actively hasten the demise of the body but also allows for the cessation of biological functioning to occur in a more natural way. This approach often allows families to feel less culpable in their loved one's death and feel they have maintained their integrity in adhering to Jewish law while caring for a family member.

## CONCLUSION

Working with diverse groups of people in challenging scenarios can require carefully developed interpersonal skills, sensitivities, and strategies. Respectful and compassionate interactions in cases such as this go a long way toward building strong relationships with the communities from which such patients come. This trust and mutual respect take time to build, and it is thus essential for medical leadership to give staff and families the time necessary to establish such rapport. The importance of striving to see things from the perspective of the other and treating them in accordance with their own goals, values, and preferences cannot be overstated and is a theme of the next chapter as we delve into the important and increasingly relevant concern of proper care for unrepresented patients.

## NOTES

1. Robert D. Troug, Wynne Morrison, and Matthew Kirschen, "What Should We Do When Families Refuse Testing for Brain Death?" *AMA Journal of Ethics* 22, no. 12 (2020): 986–94; and Ariane Lewis and David Greer, "Point: Should Informed Consent Be Required for Apnea Testing in Patients with Suspected Brain Death? No," *Chest* 152, no. 4 (2017): 700–702.

2. See, for example, discussion in John M. Luce and Ann Alpers, "Legal Aspects of Withholding and Withdrawing Life Support from Critically Ill Patients in the United States and Providing Palliative Care to Them," *American Journal of Respiratory and Critical Care Medicine* 163 (2000): 2029.

3. Thaddeus Mason Pope, "Brain Death Forsaken: Growing Conflict and New Legal Challenges," *Journal of Legal Medicine* 37 (2017): 282, 291, 294, 316.

4. Pope, 274, 277.

5. Pope, 269.

6. Eran Segal, "Religious Objections to Brain Death," *Journal of Critical Care* 29, no. 5 (2014): 875–77, https://doi.org/10.1016/j.jcrc.2014.06.017.

7. See extensive discussion on the extent to which clinicians must accommodate religious objections to brain death in Pope, "Brain Death Forsaken," 316–24.

8. Douglas A. Drossman and Johannah Ruddy, "Improving Patient-Provider Relationships to Improve Health Care," *Clinical Gastroenterology and Hepatology* 18 (2020): 1417–26.

9. A. Steinberg, *HaRefuah KeHalakhah*, vol. 6 (Jerusalem: printed by the author, 2017), 463–65.

10. Marcie Fisher-Borne, Jessie Montana Cain, and Suzanne L. Martin, "From Mastery to Accountability: Cultural Humility as an Alternative to Cultural Competence," *Social Work Education* 34, no. 2 (2015): 165–81, http://dx.doi.org/10.1080/02615479.2014.977244. Another critique of the concept of "cultural competence" argues that it reflects embedded ethnocentrism, perpetuates entrenched biases, and fails to recognize the depth and breadth of systemic racism as they relate to the mitigation of health disparities. Jeffrey T. Berger and Dana Ribeiro Miller, "Health Disparities, Systemic Racism, and Failures of Cultural Competence," *American Journal of Bioethics* 21, no. 9 (2021): 4.

11. A. Steinberg, *Encyclopedia of Jewish Medical Ethics*, vol. 3 (Jerusalem: Feldheim, 2003), 1059.

# CHAPTER SIX

# Unrepresented Patients

Having begun to deal with issues of cultural humility and mitigating conflict between patients and health care providers brings us to one of the most challenging issues in contemporary health care and medical decision-making: how to care for patients who cannot speak for themselves. While there has been much discussion related to proper care for patients who left instructions or have someone to speak on their behalf, which I will briefly review below, less has been written on caring for patients who have no one available to speak for them.[1] It is thus crucial to develop clear and rigorous guidelines to properly care for these patients. As we seek to develop approaches to guide care providers, the Jewish tradition offers a unique and important perspective for this discussion, although very little has currently been written on it from a Jewish viewpoint.

In this chapter, therefore, I present an understanding of some fundamental Jewish principles that can provide clear guidance in navigating this challenge. I then apply those values to a specific set of suggested behaviors, one of which adds an additional original component to past expert recommendations. The aim of these suggestions is not to impose Jewish values on patients but to use the Jewish tradition to help develop a new approach to a very complex and challenging area of health care. The suggested approach may be especially meaningful to Jewish practitioners or anyone working with Jewish patients.

# THE DILEMMA: INCAPACITATED PATIENTS WITH A SURROGATE

A common challenge is decision-making on behalf of incapacitated patients about whom something is known and there is a surrogate decision-maker involved (this includes those who are alert but lack decision-making capacity, such as those suffering from a severe stroke, Alzheimer's, Parkinson's, senility, or mental illness severe enough to worsen cognitive function).[2] If such a patient has not made their health care wishes known, such as through an advance directive, then a surrogate is usually asked to assist with decision-making. Family members are often turned to first because it is assumed they can be trusted to care about the patient's welfare and best interests, their long-term relationship makes them best qualified to judge what that patient would have wanted if they could respond, and they are the ones the patient would have turned to for advice.[3] However, if a family member is also unable to make reasoned judgments, doesn't have adequate knowledge of the patient, or is not committed to the patient's best interests (e.g., there is a conflict of interest), then a physician or other health care professional, institutional committee, or sometimes a court will step in to make the decisions.[4] No matter who is making the decision, whenever such decisions are made on behalf of another person, both American law and Jewish law suggest the following standards for decision-making in order of preference:[5]

1. *Advance directive*: The ideal is to attempt to respect the autonomy of the patient and follow the guidelines they have laid out in their advance directive. However, most people do not have an advance directive prepared, and even when they do, it can be difficult to find or may not provide clear guidance.[6]

2. *Substituted judgment*: Also an autonomy-based standard, the substituted judgment approach may be used if there is no instructional advance directive or if it is difficult to apply to the case at hand. In such instances, the decision-maker must attempt to determine what *the patient would have wanted* if they were competent. The surrogate decision-maker must attempt to ignore their own judgment and try to figure out what the patient would have done in that situation. The patient's intention can be inferred from prior conversations or actions of the patient or teachings from the patient's religious or moral belief system.[7]

3. *Best interests standard*: If a patient's preference is simply unknown, the decision-maker must act with beneficence to determine the highest probable benefit and whatever they think is best for the patient, or they must simply choose for the patient the actions that most people would choose.[8] This standard is also used for patients who were never competent (such as small children) or left no reliable trace of their preferences.

## UNREPRESENTED PATIENTS

The usual decision-making steps are not always possible, however. When there is no one available who is legally recognized as able to speak on behalf of an incapacitated patient, the process of making important health care decisions on their behalf is especially difficult. Making appropriate decisions for them can be excruciating, especially when virtually nothing is known about them as an individual, sometimes not even their names (an "unidentified patient"), as might occur with an individual experiencing homelessness, for example. Many American hospitals care for an alarmingly high number of these patients. They are often referred to as "adult orphans," "unbefriended," "isolated," or "incapacitated patients without advocates," but the most common term is "unrepresented."[9] Such patients currently account for over 5 percent of deaths in intensive care units, and the numbers are increasing, particularly among the elderly, homeless, and mentally disabled.[10] The situation has become even worse during the COVID-19 pandemic due to patients' confusion and isolation as a result of strict visitation policies, causing significant moral distress to clinicians.[11]

These patients are some of the most vulnerable people in our society, and since so little is known about them as individuals, making medical decisions for them is one of the most difficult and controversial challenges that arises in hospitals and bioethics today.[12] As a result, these patients are often exposed to either overtreatment, undertreatment, or delayed treatment and are likely to receive medical care that conflicts with their own preferences, values, and best interests.[13] There is no uniform decision-making standard to guide care providers in these cases, nor is there consensus on the proper procedures, and there are very few laws or policies in place to protect this population.[14]

Applying the "best interests standard" can be challenging because it is often not clear which decision is actually in a given patient's best interest. Therefore, it is ideal to strive for substituted judgment to the extent possible, even though that framework is not always clear either. However, what often happens is simply that an individual physician unilaterally makes all health care decisions with almost no oversight.[15] This situation is problematic because giving one person so much authority risks treatment plans that are not carefully thought out or are made based on a conflict of interest, such as institutional financial pressures.[16] Furthermore, studies show that physicians often simply make decisions based on their own preferences, not the patient's values.[17] This result may come about because physicians have not had the opportunity or taken the time to get to know the patient in depth, leading to possible negative assumptions, mistreatment, or treatment that is discordant with the patient's actual wishes. In addition, because physicians often rotate and each one may have different views about proper care plans, unrepresented patients may be exposed to a lack of continuity of care and further arbitrariness in treatment decisions.[18] Moral guidance is needed to support these patients and their health care providers, and although traditional Jewish law does not afford unlimited decision-making autonomy to patients, their own goals and preferences can often be relevant in determining appropriate interventions.

## JEWISH VALUES AND LAWS

Two of the most fundamental and important Jewish values may provide us with significant guidance on this issue. The Talmud teaches that Rabbi Akiva regarded "Love your neighbor as yourself" (Lev. 19:18) as the single greatest encompassing principle of the Torah. Another of the great sages, Ben Azzai, responded that the verse "This is the book of the generations of Adam" is an even more all-encompassing principle than that because this verse concludes with the idea that all humanity are created in the image of God, and degrading any person is thus akin to degrading God.[19] When fleshed out and applied to bioethics, these core values can have a deeper meaning in health care by demonstrating that more than respecting autonomy, a primary focus of interactions with patients should be the inherent duties that health care providers have to care for every individual in their care, as will be explained below.

### Love for Fellow People

The "Golden Rule" of "Love your neighbor as yourself" adds a level of personal responsibility to the bioethical ideal of substituted judgment and can serve as an important anchor for it. In addition to Rabbi Akiva referring to this commandment as the major encompassing principle of the Torah, the Talmud records that the great sage Hillel referred to it as "the entire Torah; the rest is just commentary," as he rephrased that directive into: "That which is hateful to you, do not do to your neighbor."[20] This teaching thus demands both seeking to benefit others and trying to avoid causing them harm. It is seen as a foundation for much of Jewish law relating to medical interventions (see discussion in chapter 8), such as the requirements to attempt to heal the sick; visit the sick, comfort mourners, escort the dead; and avoid infecting others.[21] It similarly bestows permission to use palliative care, and prohibits the desecration of a corpse, among many more such examples.[22]

Seeing this Golden Rule simply as treating others the way you yourself would want to be treated has led some bioethicists to critique its usefulness in clinical practice because studies have shown that when health care providers attempt to infer their patients' beliefs and desires from what they assume their own preferences would be under similar circumstances, they often make mistakes in predicting a patient's wishes or beliefs.[23] However, many classic commentaries understand this verse as a biblical obligation to show love for others in the way that you would want if you were in the other person's circumstances.[24] Some even say that this commandment is about respecting other people's autonomy by acting lovingly toward them in the way that you wish they would act lovingly toward you.[25] Everyone is different and has different needs. It is thus reasonable to assume that most people want to be treated in accordance with their own goals, values, and preferences as much as possible. This school of thought sees the Golden Rule as attempting to understand another person's own narrative, experience, beliefs, and desires. Accordingly, this verse indeed commands us to treat others not "as you would have them do unto you" but as they would have you do unto them (assuming it is not an act that violates Jewish law).[26]

Indeed, this value leads to a profound ideal in the Mishnah, which states that one of the ways the Torah is acquired is by "sharing the burden of others" (*nosei be'ol im chavero*).[27] Some of the leading thinkers of the Jewish ethics and character development movement (*mussar*) explain that this means that one must strive to do the utmost to understand and feel another person's situation from within that person's own context and life experience.[28] This commandment thus supports the need to strive to provide substituted judgment to the greatest extent possible when making decisions on behalf of unrepresented patients (see the section "Striving to Learn about Patients," below).

## Divine Image

The first ethical teaching of the Torah is the theological claim that all humans are created in the image of God (Gen. 1:26–28). This teaching imbues human beings with responsibilities and is the basis for many Torah commandments, including the prohibition against murder (Gen. 9:6), the obligation to bury the dead (Deut. 21:23), and the duty to save life.[29] Furthermore, this value leads to the category of Jewish law known as *kevod habriyot*, human dignity, which requires treating all people with basic respect and dignity.[30] This value is so crucial that concerns for protecting human dignity override much of Jewish law, particularly in order to avoid embarrassing people and preserving their reputation.[31] Although people can act in ways that betray the dignity of their image of God, or can be treated in ways that are an affront to their image of God, a person never loses their inherent image of God, even if they are incapacitated and, indeed, even after death (Deut. 21:23).[32]

Based on this understanding, the Talmudic sages created a profound ritual that is especially relevant for our discussion of caring for unrepresented patients. The Torah has certain categories of prohibitions that incur the death penalty. However, the rabbis severely limited and restricted the practical application of capital punishment. One of the ways they did so was by means of very careful examination of the witnesses in a capital case. Before giving potentially incriminating testimony, the witnesses had to be told a number of things by the court, including that "Adam was created alone to teach you that anyone who destroys one soul, the verse blames them as if they destroyed an entire world, but anyone who sustains one soul, the verse credits them as if they sustained an entire world."[33] They would then go on to tell the witnesses that

> this was done due to the importance of maintaining peace among people, so that one person cannot say to another: My progenitor is greater than yours. . . . It also tells of the greatness of God, since when a person stamps several coins with one seal, they are all similar to each other, but the supreme King of kings, the Holy Blessed One, stamped all people with the seal of Adam, the first person, yet not one of them is like another. Therefore, every person is obligated to say: "The world was created for me."[34]

This ritual reflects the view that for a witness to be relied on in life-and-death matters, they must be reminded of the tremendous import and fundamental dignity of all human life, created in the image of God. This statement can be summarized as declaring three things:[35]

- that every human life is of immeasurable value;
- that every human life is of equal value;
- that everyone is unique.[36]

This Talmudic ritual, taken to remind people of the human dignity inherent in every person but especially those most vulnerable, can serve as a model to be applied in contemporary care for unrepresented patients. Similar to those accused of crimes, whose fates are determined by a committee, every patient, no matter their condition, deserves the utmost respect and equitable treatment in accordance with their own individual values to the extent that is possible.

## STRIVING TO LEARN ABOUT PATIENTS

These values may offer useful guidance for how to approach making decisions for unrepresented patients. In order to respect the dignity and uniqueness of each person, it should not be assumed that just because a patient is unrepresented they do not have values and preferences. Most likely someone, somewhere, knows something about them.[37] So, whenever possible, there should be a diligent search to attempt to find a surrogate before making a decision.[38] Or expand the list of those who can be considered a valid surrogate in order to increase the chances of finding a person who has information about this individual's goals, values, or preferences.[39] However, it is often very difficult to locate such an individual, and at times there truly is no one available who knows a given patient.[40] Yet, even then, it may be possible to find some sort of evidence about how an individual lived their life in order to attempt to infer some of their values.[41] These Jewish principles suggest that not only is this an expectation of some contemporary bioethicists but that there may also be a biblical obligation to make every attempt to do so.

## DIVERSE INTERDISCIPLINARY DECISION-MAKING COMMITTEES

Beyond that, and particularly when nothing at all can be learned about a patient or anyone whom they might know, respect for the inherent value and dignity of each human being as well as the equality of all persons demand that hospitals develop rigorous decision-making processes for these patients in order to ensure that they are treated fairly and with dignity—not just out of respect for their autonomy but because there is an obligation to care for individuals this way.

Some states in the United States authorize clinicians to make the decision with almost no oversight, and others require the safeguard of a second physician or committee to oversee medical decisions made on behalf of unrepresented patients.[42] Yet other states have a tiered approach in which they allow an attending physician to make routine decisions alone but require approval from another physician for more risky major medical treatments, and they require consultation with an independent physician or multidisciplinary committee (or court approval) for decisions involving life-sustaining treatment.[43] Although it is essential to ensure a decision-making process that is accessible, quick, convenient, and cost effective, using the values outlined above for cases that are neither urgent nor routine would seem to require engaging in the most rigorous safeguards of expertise, neutrality, and careful deliberation.[44] I therefore believe that in decision-making for unrepresented patients, Jewish ethics would advocate for following the more demanding process of involving a diverse interdisciplinary committee, comprising not only the treating clinicians but also individuals representing that patient's own religious or cultural community whenever necessary and possible.

Indeed, in addition to the careful oversight of witnesses in capital cases in a Jewish court, the sages of the Talmud created the counterintuitive policy that if all twenty-three judges deciding on a capital case vote unanimously to convict, then the defendant goes free because complete unanimity indicates that not enough of an attempt was made to explore and understand different arguments and perspectives.[45] Using an interdisciplinary committee to carefully deliberate would thus reflect Jewish values, in that it would seek to avoid bias and conflict of interest and to safeguard procedural fairness, transparency, consistency, and oversight while ensuring that multiple, carefully weighed perspectives are incorporated.[46] This process should thus be used for complex cases even when state laws permit a far simpler standard because it offers a higher likelihood of fair and rigorous decision-making than does a single person making unilateral decisions without oversight.[47] Achieving good ethical consensus is not merely about agreement but is about who is agreeing and the quality of the deliberative process.[48]

## RITUALIZING THESE VALUES

The values detailed above encourage following the strictest standards of the bioethicists quoted in this chapter and using an interdisciplinary committee rather than simply having an individual physician unilaterally make all health care decisions. However, I believe these values require us to go even further and take steps to ritualize these ideals, based on the formal statement about the image of God read to witnesses in capital cases, mentioned above. Busy schedules and the high volume of these sorts of cases may unfortunately lead to some practitioners occasionally forgetting that an unidentified patient is more than just a body lying in a hospital bed. Even when a practitioner values something, research has shown that an act of "priming," which is simply reading a statement or being reminded of one's values prior to being asked to engage in an act, increases the likelihood of compliance with one's own values and keeping their positive intentions in mind.[49] I therefore recommend that prior to meeting to make medical decisions on behalf of unrepresented patients, a brief formal statement should be read, reminding each participant of the value, equality, and uniqueness of every human being, modeled after the Talmudic statement made to witnesses in capital cases, in order to protect highly vulnerable populations. Ideally this statement should include the patient's name and sharing some known detail about them or displaying a photo of them, if possible. This statement should be as inclusive as possible and refer to the extent of the health care provider's duty to care for others and to provide care that is as concordant with the patient's own goals and values as possible, highlighting the dignity of each person and the magnitude of the decisions being made on their behalf.

In the diverse health care environment, this statement could be something as simple as reading aloud an inclusive and nonsectarian line such as, "Before engaging in making decisions on behalf of this patient (insert name if known), we hereby recognize their inherent value and uniqueness and commit ourselves to striving to understand who they are, to fulfill our duties toward them, and care for them equitably and with dignity to the best of our ability."

In the Jewish tradition, ritual practices, such as the Passover seder, are frequently used to help transform abstract ideals into living practices that shape character.[50] Similar types of priming statements are made before performing many mitzvot (biblical commandments). For example, some traditional Jewish prayer books suggest beginning one's day by proclaiming, "I hereby take upon myself to fulfill the commandment to 'love your fellow person as yourself.'"[51] So, too, the idea of health care providers engaging in helpful rituals is not unheard of in contemporary health care.[52] For example, many emergency rooms and intensive care units have implemented "post-code pauses" (also known as "post-resuscitation debriefings") in which, following a resuscitation, trauma, or death, staff engage in a formalized moment of silence, followed by some simple reflections, questions, and debriefing in order to pay homage to the patient and process their own thoughts and feelings before continuing their shift.[53] These pauses have been shown to help health care providers feel more present and able to meet the needs of all of their patients.[54]

## CONCLUSION

Although Jewish ethics reaches many of the same conclusions as some of the most rigorous standards put forward in secular bioethics, these conclusions come from different starting points, which add additional insights and responsibilities. Most bioethicists who write on the topic of making decisions for incapacitated patients base their models primarily on respect for the patient's autonomy.[55] This Jewish approach focuses less on patients' rights and more on care providers' obligations to care for them and to protect their intrinsic dignity, which can have a significant impact on how and why decisions are made.[56] After all, being created in the image of God not only confers human dignity but also means that our lives belong to God and thus that our own autonomy is not the primary value.[57] This duty-based perspective requires a very high threshold of striving to ensure that the right thing be done, in the right way, and that we develop a society in which everyone can rely on being protected when they are most vulnerable.[58] Basing such decisions on these universal biblical values and ideology can serve to heighten care providers' sensitivity to treating each patient with dignity and their sense of obligation to do so. Moreover, ritualizing this process and verbalizing these values adds an additional reminder that can help ensure that they are in fact acted upon on a regular basis.

All that said, there are times in contemporary medicine in which health care providers' moral distress is stretched to the limit. What options one has when they object to things they witness in a hospital or to interventions that they are asked to participate in, and how far one should or should not go in objecting, are the subject of the next chapter.

## NOTES

1. David Godfrey, "Health Care Decision-Making during a Crisis When Nothing Is in Writing," *National Academy of Elder Law Attorneys Journal* 15 (2019): 1–16.

2. Tom L. Beauchamp and James F. Childress, *Principles of Biomedical Ethics*, 8th ed. (New York: Oxford University Press, 2019), 139–42.

3. Benjamin Freedman, *Duty and Healing: Foundations of a Jewish Bioethic* (New York: Routledge, 1999), 77; Beauchamp and Childress, *Principles of Biomedical Ethics*, 195; and *Iggerot Moshe*, CM 2:74:5.

4. Beauchamp and Childress, *Principles of Biomedical Ethics*, 195.

5. On American law, see Beauchamp and Childress, 226–28. On Jewish law, see the extensive discussion in Jason Weiner, *Jewish Guide to Practical Medical Decision-Making* (Jerusalem: Urim, 2017), chap. 2B.

6. Thaddeus Mason Pope, "Unbefriended and Unrepresented: Better Medical Decision Making for Incapacitated Patients without Healthcare Surrogates," *Georgia State University Law Review* 33, no. 4 (2017): 935–36.

7. Pope, 939–40, 1003.

8. H. Schacter, *BeIkvei HaTzon*, 34.

9. Pope, "Unbefriended and Unrepresented," 925; and Thaddeus Mason Pope, Joshua Bennett, Shannon S. Carson, Lynette Cederquist, Andrew B. Cohen, Erin S. DeMartino, David M. Godfrey, et al., "Making Medical Treatment Decisions for Unrepresented Patients in the ICU: An Official American Thoracic Society/American Geriatrics Society Policy Statement," *American Journal of Respiratory and Critical Care Medicine* 201, no. 10 (2020): 1183; and David Ozar, "Who Are 'Unrepresented' Patients and What Count as 'Important Medical Decisions' for Them?" *AMA Journal of Ethics* 21, no. 7 (2019): 611. For an excellent working definition of "unrepresented patient," see p. 613.

10. Scott J. Schweikart, "Who Makes Decisions for Incapacitated Patients Who Have No Surrogate or Advance Directive?" *AMA Journal of Ethics* 21, no. 7 (2019): 587–93.

11. Krishna Chokshi, "The Burden of Deciding for Others: Caring for Unrepresented Patients with COVID-19," *Voices in Bioethics* 6 (2020), https://doi.org/10.7916/vib.v6i.7224.

12. Pope, "Unbefriended and Unrepresented," 925.

13. Pope, 953; and Thaddeus Mason Pope, "Five Things Clinicians Should Know When Caring for Unrepresented Patients," *AMA Journal of Ethics* 21, no. 7 (2019): 582–83. Unfortunately, this is also often the case even with patients who have surrogates, since surrogates frequently make mistakes about what the patients would have actually wanted. Bruce Jennings, ed., *Encyclopedia of Bioethics*, 4th ed. (Macmillan Reference, 2014), 6:3038.

14. Pope, "Unbefriended and Unrepresented," 928.

15. Douglas B. White, J. Randall Curtis, Bernard Lo, and John M. Luce, "Decisions to Limit Life-Sustaining Treatment for Critically Ill Patients Who Lack Both Decision-Making Capacity and Surrogate Decision-Makers," *Critical Care Medicine* 34, no. 8 (2006): 2053–59.

16. Pope, "Unbefriended and Unrepresented," 986–89, 991.

17. Pope, 955, 990.

18. Ozar, "Who Are 'Unrepresented' Patients?" 612.

19. *Sifra*, *Kedoshim* 4:12; and Jerusalem Talmud, *Nedarim* 32a (chap. 9, halakhah 4), with explanation of *Pnei Moshe* and *Korban HaEidah*. See also *Daat Zekeinim* on Genesis 5:1 and *Michtav MeEliyahu* 3, p. 90. Some thus argue that Ben Azzai is not actually disagreeing with Rabbi Akiva but rather giving the reason for the obligation to love one's neighbor as themselves and broadening the requirement to all of humanity. See discussion in David Novak, *Covenantal Rights: A Study in Jewish Political Theory* (Princeton, NJ: Princeton University Press, 2000), 148–49.

20. *Shabbat* 31a.

21. On attempting to heal the sick, see Ramban, *Torat HaAdam Sha'ar HaSakanah*, s.v. *aval rabbeinu*; and *Tzitz Eliezer* 5: *Ramat Rachel*, 21. See also further discussion in *Encyclopedia Hilkhatit Refu'it*, 7, 178, and 5, 681. On visiting the sick, comforting mourners, and escorting the dead, see Rambam, *Hilkhot Avel*, 14:1. On avoiding infecting others, see *Sefer Chassidim*, 673, which says that, based on the verse "Love your neighbor as yourself," one who has a skin disease may not bathe with another person without informing them first.

22. Rabbi S. Z. Auerbach argues that alleviating pain falls under the obligation to love one's neighbor as oneself. Responsa *Minchat Shlomo* 2–3:86. Rabbi M. Shteinberg writes that the prohibition of desecrating the dead is not just part of the obligation to bury the dead

but is based on the verse "Love your neighbor as yourself" and thus permits "desecrating" the dead, such as with an autopsy, when it is being done in order to save a life or even for money for the surviving family or if the deceased gave permission to do so when they were alive. *Noam 3*, 95 based on *Sanhedrin* 45a and *Ritva, Makkot* 7; see also *Encyclopedia Hilkhatit Refu'it*, 5, 596; and *Tzitz Eliezer* 4:14.

23. Sunil Kothari and Kristi L. Kirschner, "Abandoning the Golden Rule: The Problem with 'Putting Ourselves in the Patient's Place,'" *Topics in Stroke Rehabilitation* 13, no. 4 (2006): 68–73.

24. Sforno, *Vayikra* 19:18, writes, "You should desire for your neighbor that which you would desire/love for yourself, were you in his position." See also *Sefer HaMitzvot*, Positive Mitzvah 206. To the Sforno and Rambam, the focus is more on achieving piety than it is on specific actions.

25. Bekhor Shor, *Vayikra* 19:18. To the Bekhor Shor, the commandment is focused specifically on duties and actions (or avoidance of certain actions) more than it is on achieving pious emotions or views of others. I would like to thank Rabbi A. Klapper for pointing out this source to me and its distinction from the Sforno, quoted in the previous note.

26. Some refer to this formulation as the "Platinum Rule" ("treat your neighbor the way they wish to be treated"), which was first articulated by Karl R. Popper, *The Open Society and Its Enemies*, vol. 2, *Hegel and Marx* (London: Routledge & Kegan Paul, 1945), 386. However, many prefer to see it as part and parcel of the expansive view of the traditional rabbinic commentaries on the Golden Rule because many thinkers have argued that the "Platinum Rule" risks misconstruing the clear meaning of the Golden Rule by focusing only on giving people whatever they want, such as providing a drug addict with more drugs if they say that's what they want, which would be problematic. Leonard Swidler, "The 'Golden Rule': The 'Best Rule,'" *Journal of Ecumenical Studies* 54, no. 1 (2019): 281. Some also generally refer to this type of thought as "Care Ethics," which is the obligation to care for the other in his or her particularity, attempting to see the world from *the other's* perspective, not merely as a sympathizer would see it. Ruth E. Groenhout, "I Can't Say No: Self-Sacrifice and an Ethics of Care," in *Philosophy, Feminism, and Faith*, ed. Ruth E. Groenhout and Marya Bower (Bloomington: Indiana University Press, 2003), 153; and Stephanie Collins, *The Core of Care Ethics* (New York: Palgrave, 2015), 24. I thank Rabbi Dr. S. Held for sharing these texts on care ethics with me.

27. *Avot* 6:6. Rabbi S. Kluger writes that this idea of "sharing the burden of others" is an outgrowth of the Torah's commandment to "love your neighbor as yourself." *Magen Avot* 6:6, also quoted in *Oz VeHadar Pirkei Avot* 6, *Kaftor VaFerach*, 90. Rabbi Y. Levovitz argues that it is not just a derivative of the Torah's commandment to "love your neighbor as yourself" but an extension of it and the very basis of Torah and mitzvot. *Da'at Chokhmah UMussar* 4, 29–32.

28. See *Chokhmah UMussar* 1, #1 and 99; *Ohr Rabbi Simcha Zissel* (Kfar Chabad, 5721), 19.

29. *Tzitz Eliezer* 17:66(7); and Cherlow, *In His Image*, 108. On responsibilities, see Yuval Cherlow, *In His Image: The Image of God in Man* (New Milford, CT: Maggid, 2015), 6. On the Torah commandments, see Joseph Soloveitchik, *Yemei Zikaron* (Jerusalem: World Zionist Organization, 1986), 9; and Cherlow, *In His Image*, 94–96, 110–13, 119.

30. That *kevod habriyot* (human dignity) is based on *Tzelem Elokim* (image of God), see

*Divrei Yosher* on *Pirkei Avot* 1:12; Ahron Soloveichik, *Logic of the Heart, Logic of the Mind: Wisdom and Reflections on Topics of Our Times* (Jerusalem: Genesis Jerusalem Press, 1991), 61; and Soloveitchik, *Yemei Zikaron*, 9. See discussion and more citations in Daniel Feldman, *The Right and the Good: Halakhah and Human Relations* (Brooklyn, NY: Yashar, 2005), 199; as well as Cherlow, *In His Image*, 122; and *Tzitz Eliezer* 17:39(2). "All people" means not just Jews. Classic Jewish sources argue that every human being equally deserves to be treated with basic respect and dignity under this category. See, for example, Responsa *Hitorerut Teshuvah* 1:75, which argues that this is also the view of the Rambam, in *Hilkhot Sanhedrin* 24:9; Soloveichik, *Logic of the Heart*, 61; Rabbi Aharon Lichtenstein, "Kevod habriyot," *Machanayim Journal* (Israel: Chief Rabbinate of the IDF, 1973), 5:8–15; and Rabbi Yitzchak Zilberstein, *Chashukei Chemed, Sanhedrin* (Israel: printed by the author, 1990), 55a. See discussion and other citations in Feldman, *Right and the Good*, 199.

31. *Berakhot* 19b–20a; *Shabbat* 81b and 94a; *Megillah* 3b; and *Eiruvin* 41b.

32. Some Jewish approaches to military ethics raise the issue of people behaving in a manner that betrays their inherent image of God to such an extent that they become unworthy of this defense, although they also argue that even one's adversary nevertheless retains their image of God, which entails restrictions on ways in which they may be attacked. Cherlow, *In His Image*, 107. *Tzitz Eliezer* 13:89 mentions that not allowing people to die in a dignified manner but rather utilizing ineffective, invasive treatments, including many tubes coming in and out of the person, may be seen by some as an affront to the patient's godly image. It is clear that Jewish values regard all people as retaining their divine image no matter what they do, from the fact that the Torah says that even the body of one convicted of murder must be buried quickly because that person is also created in the image of God (Deut. 21:23). See discussion in Cherlow, *In His Image*, 104. On incapacitation, see, for example, A. Steinberg, *HaRefuah KeHalakhah*, vol. 2 (Jerusalem: printed by the author, 2017), 158, who makes this point by arguing that according to the Torah, a baby is considered to be in the image of God, as are adults who do not possess intellectual or decision-making capacity or even the ability to think, whereas a robot or computer that can process information and speak is not considered to be created in the image of God.

33. This translation is based on the Jerusalem Talmud, *Sanhedrin* (chap. 4, halakhah 9) and earlier manuscripts of the Babylonian Talmud (such as the Munich and the Genizah manuscripts) as well as the early Mishnah manuscripts (such as Kaufman and Cambridge) and *Pirkei DeRabbi Eliezer* (Hager); *Chorev* 47; *Tanna DeVei Eliyahu Rabbah* (Ish Shalom), 11; Rambam, *Sanhedrin* 12:3, which all read "one soul," as quoted here. Adam is regarded by the Torah as the progenitor of all humans, not only Jews, so this inclusive universal reading of the text is logical. Michael Rosensweig, "Reflections on Racism and Social Divisiveness," *Tradition* 53, no. 2 (Spring 2021): 7. See also *Mashiv Milchamah* 1:1 and sources quoted in footnote 30 above.

34. *Sanhedrin* 37a.

35. Jonathan Sacks, *Covenant & Conversation, a Weekly Reading of the Jewish Bible: Numbers* (New Milford, CT: Maggid, 2017), 230; H. Yoskowitz, *Health Care and Holiness: A Jewish View* (Collegeville, MN: Jay Phillips Chair in Jewish Studies, 1995), 2; and Irving Greenberg, *The Triumph of Life* (forthcoming), chap. 2.

36. Some prefer to say that life is of "infinite value"; see, for example, discussion in Levi

Meier, *Jewish Values in Health and Medicine* (Lanham, MD: University Press of America, 1991), 60. However, many rabbinic scholars and philosophers argue that referring to human life as "infinite" is inaccurate because that would imply that everything possible must be done at all times to prolong every moment of life, no matter how much pain or costs are involved, which is not always the case. See the extensive discussion in Weiner, *Jewish Guide to Practical Medical Decision-Making*, 39–41.

37. Cynthia Griggins, Eric Blackstone, Lauren McAliley, and Barbara Daly, "Making Medical Decisions for Incapacitated Patients without Proxies: Part I," *HEC Forum* 32 (2020): 33–45, https://doi.org/10.1007/s10730-019-09387-3.

38. Pope, "Unbefriended and Unrepresented," 956, 962–63.

39. Pope, 964–67.

40. Pope, 972, 977.

41. Pope et al., "Making Medical Treatment Decisions," 1189.

42. Pope et al., 1190; and Pope, "Unbefriended and Unrepresented," 991.

43. Pope, 999–1002.

44. Pope, 1018; and Ozar, "Who Are 'Unrepresented' Patients?" 614.

45. *Sanhedrin*, 17a; *Mishneh Torah, Sanhedrin* 9:1; *Maharatz Chiyut, Sanhedrin* 17a; and *Arukh HaShulchan*, CM 18:7.

46. For example, explaining the importance of engaging different perspectives, the *Tiferet Yisrael* on *Avot* 5:17 argues that "it is through differences of opinion and back and forth discussions on each side that truth becomes clarified." See also Pope et al., "Making Medical Treatment Decisions," 1189. Although this process has more administrative burdens, takes time, and could lead to group think, these problems can be overcome if carried out responsibly, and the disadvantages are outweighed by the importance of maintaining procedural fairness and the particularity of each patient.

47. Pope et al., "Making Medical Treatment Decisions," 1190.

48. See, for example, Jonathan D. Moreno, *Deciding Together: Bioethics and Moral Consensus* (New York: Oxford University Press, 1995).

49. See, for example, the positive impact "priming" has been shown to have on vaccine compliance in Noel T. Brewer, Gretchen B. Chapman, Alexander J. Rothman, Julie Leask, and Allison Kempe, "Increasing Vaccination: Putting Psychological Science into Action," *Psychological Science in the Public Interest* 18, no. 3 (2017): 178; and regarding hand hygiene in hospitals, in Dominic King, Ivo Vlaev, Ruth Everett-Thomas, Maureen Fitzpatrick, Ara Darzi, and David J Birnbach, "'Priming' Hand Hygiene Compliance in Clinical Environments," *Health Psychology* 35, no. 1 (2016): 96–101.

50. *Sefer HaChinuch*, #606; and Jonathan Sacks, *To Heal a Fractured World: The Ethics of Responsibility* (New York: Schocken, 2005), 171.

51. *Siddur Tehillat Hashem, Nusach HaAri Zal*, beginning of morning prayers right before "*Mah Tovu*" (see *Magen Avraham*, OH 46:1). Similarly, Rabbi J. Sacks argues that the daily morning blessings recited at the beginning of Jewish prayer books are intended "to make us conscious of what we might otherwise take for granted. Praise is an act of focused attention, foregrounding what is usually in the background of awareness." Jonathan Sacks, *The Koren Siddur* (Jerusalem: Koren Publishers, 2009), 27.

52. Indeed, in the early days of bioethics consultations, some suggested that meetings among health care providers to discuss goals of care should be conceptualized as the ritual of a "Greek chorus" to ensure that decisions are not made hastily or arbitrarily; see Kathryn Montgomery Hunter, "Limiting Treatment in a Social Vacuum: A Greek Chorus for William T," *Archives of Internal Medicine* 145, no. 4 (1985): 716–19.

53. Darcy Copeland and Heather Liska, "Implementation of a Post-Code Pause: Extending Post-Event Debriefing to Include Silence," *Journal of Trauma Nursing* 23, no. 2 (2016): 58–64.

54. Tim Cunningham, Dallas M. Ducar, and Jessica Keim-Malpass, "'The Pause': A Delphi Methodology Examining an End-of-Life Practice," *Western Journal of Nursing Research* 41, no. 10 (2019): 1481–98.

55. See, for example, Beauchamp and Childress, *Principles of Biomedical Ethics*, 139–42; Lisa Soleymani Lehman, "Family Dynamics and Surrogate Decision-Making," in *Guidance for Healthcare Ethics Committees*, ed. D. Micah Hester and Toby Schonfeld (Cambridge: Cambridge University Press, 2012), 64; and Pope, "Unbefriended and Unrepresented," 931.

56. Freedman, *Duty and Healing*, 98.

57. Sacks, *To Heal a Fractured World*, 167.

58. Sacks, 128–29. Laurie Zoloth refers to this as taking "responsibility for responsibility." Laurie Zoloth, *Second Texts / Second Opinions: Essays toward a Jewish Bioethics* (Oxford: Oxford University Press, 2022), chap. 9.

# CHAPTER SEVEN

# Conscientious Objection

Most medical professionals are guided primarily by their own deeply held morals and values, not what their professional organizations require of them.[1] Some health care providers do not feel comfortable participating in certain interventions that go against their personal core values. As medicine achieves the ability to accomplish more, interventions become available that present increasing challenges. Refusal to participate in these interventions is known as "conscientious objection," which has been defined as "the rejection of some action by a provider, primarily because the action would violate some deeply held moral or ethical value about right and wrong."[2]

The issue of conscientious objection is ancient, finding expression in Jewish biblical values.[3] It arose in modern medicine when some physicians refused to comply with abusive forms of medicine forced onto a population by totalitarian regimes, as was the case in Nazi Germany.[4] It continues to be relevant in contemporary health care settings in terms of the participation of health care professionals, such as doctors, nurses, and pharmacists in certain procedures, including euthanasia, physician aid in dying, contraception, and other reproductive technologies. Following the 1973 *Roe v. Wade* abortion decision, the United States Congress passed "conscience clause" legislation, known as the "Church Amendment," which protected an individual's right of refusal to take part in abortion and sterilization (42 U.S.C. 300a-7).[5] This amendment prohibited courts and government agencies from requiring individuals or facilities to perform abortions or sterilizations if they had moral objections and protected individuals from employer discrimination if they were unwilling to perform abortions or sterilizations.[6]

Such legislation has not been without controversy, and several states, as well as many countries, have taken extremely divergent approaches.[7] The debate surrounding the appropriateness of health care providers engaging in conscientious objection has been intense and often polarizing. This chapter summarizes various arguments in the bioethical literature, both favoring and opposing conscientious objection; offers some proposed solutions; and then presents a paradigm-shifting compromise approach that arises out of very recent Jewish bioethical thought.

## ARGUMENTS IN FAVOR OF
## CONSCIENTIOUS OBJECTION

While some argue that conscientious objection is a matter of freedom to practice one's religion, most feel that the foundation for exercising this right is even more fundamental.[8] Many contend that a multicultural and tolerant society should simply not be attempting to impose ethical beliefs on others but rather should strive to accept various moral viewpoints. They thus see respect for conscientious objection as a form of tolerance for "moral diversity."[9] Similarly, others argue that conscientious objection is a type of ethical modesty or humility because it recognizes that one might be mistaken and should thus not be dogmatic regarding differing viewpoints.[10] To obligate one to go against their religious or ethical convictions is also regarded as a form of discrimination and a violation of ethical and human rights.[11] Some even see conscientious objection as being integral to a functioning democracy. They suggest that just as people should have the essential right to object to being drafted into military service, they should also have the right to refuse to engage in behaviors they see as immoral.[12]

However, what a professional can object to is limited, and some things cannot be tolerated, such as unnecessarily violating patient confidentiality or engaging in discrimination, based on race, sexual orientation, and so on.[13] Some thus claim that it is the principle of respect for autonomy that is the strongest basis for both a patient's right to refuse treatments and a clinician's right not to engage in them.[14] Respect for individual autonomy implies that professionals should not have to abandon their morals in order to get a job, or to leave their job if new interventions become required of them, and that individuals should be allowed to select which procedures they are comfortable participating in as part of a right to free choice of employment.[15] Just as reproductive rights and abortion are often seen as matters of personal choice, so should a professional have a choice *not* to participate.[16]

Beyond autonomy arguments, many thinkers frame the importance of conscientious objection as most fundamentally respecting the need of individuals to maintain their "moral integrity."[17] This formulation allows health care providers to see themselves not only as technicians, like auto mechanics, but recognizes that someone who engages in procedures that go against their conscience and violate their own morality will feel that they are not being true to themselves.[18] Such moral distress can cause a loss of self-respect and may lead to burnout, fatigue, and emotional exhaustion.[19] In addition to such possible negative implications, some claim that a professional only becomes and remains a responsible moral agent through a gradual process of observation, reflection, and practice, which must be protected so that it can develop.[20]

From this perspective, protecting the moral integrity of health care professionals can benefit the entire society since many people would want to have their own morality and integrity respected, and everyone benefits from having medical professionals who are trustworthy and honest moral public servants. Such behavior would not be promoted if professionals were asked to forsake their ethics in some situations yet apply them to patient welfare in other areas.[21] Moreover, allowing students and residents conscience-based exemptions might increase their ethical sensitivity.[22] Protection of moral integrity and a health care professional's right to refuse to participate thus promotes the common good as it enables society to benefit from professionals who are encouraged to practice with these virtues.[23] Some also make the case that allowing practitioners to set limits on the interventions they are morally comfortable performing allows health care professionals to practice their vocation with individual integrity and thus earn their patients' trust.[24] While some will argue that the public good is ultimately not served by restricting access to health care, if other providers are willing to offer such services without excessive burden to the patient, a pluralistic society is better served by respecting the interests of as many individuals' rights as possible—both those in search of these services and those who do not want to engage in them.[25]

## ARGUMENTS AGAINST CONSCIENTIOUS OBJECTION

Principled opposition has arisen to the idea that medical professionals should have a right to conscientious objection. One example is the "incompatibility thesis," which maintains that medical professionals voluntarily join a profession that is expected to serve society by providing essential services, all of which are legal and professionally accepted, and refusing to do so is incompatible with

their professional responsibilities.[26] From this perspective, medical professionals have an obligation to use their skills to serve their patients, placing the interests of their patients above their own (often referred to as "patient-centered
care"). Furthermore, since they have freely chosen this field—unlike a military
draft—some would argue that they must adopt its obligations.[27] Those who
take this approach argue that individuals should not go into a line of work in
which they are conflicted and unable to carry out all of its professional expectations, and particularly not a specialty that includes procedures one is unwilling
to engage in.[28]

From this perspective, although everyone is entitled to have their own values
in their private lives, some see medical professionals as public servants who
should thus minimize the extent to which their own values impact communal
interests.[29] Moreover, allowing conscientious objection places burdens on patients and compromises their care by lowering the quality of health care.[30] This
is because it can render health care inconsistent since treatment can become
dependent on the values of a given doctor, and inefficient, since people must
search for doctors who are willing to provide the services they need.[31] Limiting
patient choice may be less detrimental to patients who have access to many
options, but it disproportionately impacts the poor, those living in rural areas,
and those with limited mobility.[32] Conscientious objection thus raises social
justice concerns since it can negatively impact the health of the most vulnerable,
which is unfair, unjust, and unnecessarily exposes them to risk. Societal needs
should therefore override individual practitioners' personal, religious, or moral
needs. If practitioners gain more opportunities to refuse treatments, they argue,
the potential for various forms of discrimination and misuse of this right will
increase.[33]

Many thinkers reject the conflation of conscientious objection with morality
and its contribution to a just society. They argue that both negative duties and
positive duties and claims of conscience exist. Therefore, just as many speak of
a refusal to engage in a given procedure as conscientious objection, those who
believe in providing such services often do so out of a commitment to core ethical beliefs, which can frame their practice as "conscientious provision."[34] From
this perspective, moral integrity can also be injured by *not* allowing an action
required by one's core commitments, just as performing an action that con-
tradicts those beliefs can cause moral injury for others. A focus on protecting
conscientious objection can thus stigmatize those in need of services as well as
those who provide them and can therefore undermine virtue and commitment
to moral ideals in society.[35]

## SOLUTIONS

While these different perspectives may seem to make much of this issue unresolvable, there are some middle-ground approaches that have been offered. The consensus is that some limits on conscientious objection may be appropriate.[36] One suggestion is that interventions for which conscientious objection may be requested should be limited, only allowing those with direct participation to object as well as requiring objectors to satisfy certain tests of genuineness, reasonableness, or rationality before being permitted to refuse involvement.[37]

Broader support exists for requiring steps to ensure that conscientious objection has minimal negative impact on the quality, efficiency, and equitability of health care. To achieve that goal, many feel that health care providers should, at a minimum,

- offer emergency lifesaving services when no alternative is available;[38]
- clearly inform patients and employers well in advance of what services they would not be willing to perform;[39] and
- never obstruct access to health care and ideally provide other options to receive those services, including respectfully providing information, options, or a timely referral.[40]

Many conscientious objectors are unwilling to provide referrals for services that they morally object to, although some have found ways to make indirect referrals.[41] Some argue that when making referrals for procedures one is unwilling to perform, providers should pay for the increased costs their patients may incur, and others suggest that those unwilling to provide these minimal accommodations should be disciplined.[42]

## JEWISH APPROACH

Rabbinic thinkers have dealt with this question, and new approaches have been offered in recent years. While much of the above comes out of Christian—especially Catholic—opposition to engage in certain medical interventions, traditional Jewish law has many of the same concerns but offers a unique perspective that frames this conscientious objection differently and can potentially provide a very helpful compromise approach for conflicted practitioners.

The way conscientious objection becomes categorized in Jewish law takes the focus away from practitioners' own moral commitments and focuses on the results of one's actions. Jewish law forbids an observant Jew from transgressing the Torah and includes some rabbinic prohibitions that serve as safeguards but are not required as strictly as biblical prohibitions. The question Jewish law asks is how concerned must one who observes Jewish law be when other people seek their support in doing something that violates Jewish law, and what biblical verse or category of rabbinic law does this fall under? Rabbinic authorities have placed the prohibition against taking part in another person's forbidden action under the category of the biblical prohibition against placing a stumbling block before the blind (Lev. 19:14). By categorizing conscientious objection this way, Jewish law can permit practitioners to do things like provide referrals and engage in ancillary support such as anesthesiology for most interventions, including those that biblical law prohibits, if the action is going to happen anyway.

This is because traditional rabbinic commentaries have understood this verse not only to be about actually tripping a blind person but also to contain two fundamental prohibitions that take "blindness" more metaphorically:

1. This verse prohibits giving bad advice to a person who is "blind" in a certain matter or to the consequences of that advice (i.e., informational blindness).[43]

2. The verse also prohibits giving someone the means, causing, or facilitating an opportunity for them to stumble morally by transgressing the Torah.[44]

The Talmud and most medieval commentators focus primarily on this second, more expansive prohibition, which leads to much concern in Jewish law about the ramifications of one's actions and, hence, the results-based categorization of conscientious objection in Jewish legal sources. The classic example in the Talmud is a prohibition against giving a cup of wine to a person who has vowed not to drink wine (a *nazir*), since giving them the cup can enable them to transgress their vow by drinking from it.[45]

While enabling sin is prohibited by this verse, this prohibition also has some crucial limits that are relevant for medical professionals. Most significantly, the Talmud rules that this commandment is violated only when the person extending the forbidden item and the person receiving it are located on two opposite sides of a river, which completely separates them, such that the person who is "morally stumbling" would be physically unable to access the forbidden item but for the assistance of the other person. Extending the forbidden item across the river places a "stumbling block" by creating the opportunity to sin and is thus prohibited by this verse.[46] However, one would not violate this verse by passing a cup to the person if both of them are on the same side of the river, meaning that the transgressor could have engaged in that prohibited action on their own without any help specifically from the one who passed the cup to them.[47] This ruling reconceptualizes the conscientious objection discussion by claiming that if a problematic action is going to occur anyway, then assisting with it is not as morally problematic.

Since enabling one to sin who could do so anyway without them (i.e., "same side of the river") does not transgress the narrow definition of the biblical prohibition, a medical professional would not be required by this biblical law to object to participating in any procedure that they may regard as immoral as long as the patient would still be able to receive it even without their involvement. However, the discussion does not end there, because the rabbis of the Talmud nevertheless prohibit that action under a category known as *mesaye'a* or "assisting" the sin of another.[48] This thus becomes the primary focus of many of those who analyze conscientious objection from a Jewish legal perspective: What actions are prohibited because they assist another person in engaging in a transgression of Jewish law and which may one assist others with, even if they would not be comfortable with it for themselves? However, rabbinic authorities can maneuver this question with much flexibility since it is categorized as a rabbinic prohibition and not a biblical one, which lowers the degree of prohibition and allows numerous other leniencies to be considered, rendering such "assistance" permissible in certain circumstances.

For example, within this rabbinic prohibition against "assisting," the rabbis permit assisting the person who is assisting the transgressor since the Torah only forbids placing a stumbling block before the blind but not placing it before another person who will then place it before the blind.[49] This principle thus allows involvement in indirect actions. In these situations, where one can transgress without the assistance of another, many argue that the prohibition only applies if assistance is directly requested and provided at the precise moment of the transgression but not if it takes place prior to the forbidden action.[50] This is a very relevant ruling when it comes to behaviors such as providing referrals or information. Some are also lenient if a prohibition is only violated by inaction, such as passively allowing prohibited actions to take place.[51] So, too, if one's livelihood depends on their professional duties, the rabbis do not require sacrificing that in order not to assist with a transgression that will be done anyway without them.[52]

The permissive category within these laws that may be the most relevant for medical professionals focuses on the claim that the reason the rabbis prohibited one from assisting another person's violation of Jewish law, even when that person can transgress on their own, is because they wanted people to discourage others from sinning. However, if the person who is sinning doesn't observe Jewish law, or knows exactly what they are doing and has decided to do the forbidden act without concern for any Torah prohibition that might exist, the rabbis did not require one to try to prevent them from doing so, and therefore this rabbinic prohibition against assisting them doesn't apply.[53] This is especially true if allowing a person to engage in a prohibited act might prevent that person from violating an even worse prohibition instead. Similarly, if one's assistance allows others to violate a lesser prohibition, one is then required to consider the long-term consequences and favor actions that will lead to less overall sin.[54] This likely applies to most situations of conscientious objection today, when patients turn to medical professionals for a desired intervention but not their moral perspective on the matter.

While not all contemporary rabbinic authorities accept this approach, many do, and its ramifications for the conscientious objection discussion are profound.[55] Although these principles arise specifically out of Jewish law, perhaps this "two sides of the river" paradigm discussed above provides a different way to look at religious objection and can be incorporated by many health care professionals. Following this approach would mean that a medical professional could, or perhaps *should*, be involved in most aspects of patient care for a patient who has decided to engage in an action that the medical professional would otherwise object to since if one professional does not do it, there are others who will. Jewish law thus permits a medical professional to be involved in any service or procedure that the patient will be able to receive anyway, without their participation, if their assistance is indirect and does not directly violate Jewish law at the moment any transgression occurs.

Framed this way, one need not see this as a compromise of their values but rather a recognition of the fact that people have options. Not only is voicing conscientious objections not always effective, it could have counterproductive consequences and lead to more sinning than less. For example, research related to physician aid in dying has shown that, paradoxically, a nonjudgmental, supportive approach from clergy has been more effective in allowing patients to consider alternatives to aid in dying, and even to ultimately change their minds, than active opposition to the patient's decision.[56] Studies have also shown that when clinicians take the time to listen compassionately to their patients and explore the reason(s) for their requests, that act of simply listening to the patients' concerns helps to mitigate many of them.[57] Similarly, regarding abortion, many women who don't have access to legal services end up attempting to abort the fetus themselves in very dangerous and even fatal ways.[58]

Therefore, as long as the medical professional is not directly performing the prohibited intervention themself, Jewish law often permits a medical professional's involvement with what could be considered "immoral" interventions, such as

- writing prescriptions;[59]
- sharing information/describing various options with a patient or making direct and effective referrals to other providers;[60]
- serving on a board that permits abortions or other such procedures;[61]
- writing DNR orders;[62]
- enrolling and caring for a patient in hospice;[63]
- administering anesthesia or other types of supportive care for abortion or other controversial procedures;[64] and
- providing marital therapy for a couple in a union forbidden by Jewish law.[65]

## CONCLUSION

I have outlined a perspective that teaches that one does not place a stumbling block when their assistance does not directly induce more sin. Indeed, objecting can become an exercise in futility or potentially cause even worse outcomes than might ensue by refusing to participate. In particular, when the individual planning to commit an act that the professional sees as immoral will not be swayed by the protest, and the act can be carried out in any event without that individual provider, we can invoke the "same side of the river" paradigm that arises out of Talmudic law. Rather than focusing specifically on the practitioner's own conscience, a practitioner can then justify taking part in most interventions. In this way, one can maintain their moral integrity even without engaging in conscientious objection while resting assured that they have not actually placed a stumbling block before the blind. It remains important to protect moral diversity, practitioners' integrity, and allow conscientious objection in some cases, but it need not be invoked nearly as frequently as it currently is. Those who believe that it is important for religious individuals, or anyone with a strong set of moral principles, to be fully involved in health care so that they can take culturally and religiously sensitive care of patients and have a positive impact on the way medical care is seen and provided in our society must find ways of working within the system.[66] Otherwise, they might be forced to simply leave some of the most crucial interventions only to those who do not share their values.

The practice of medicine affords a profound privilege for medical professionals to have a positive impact on many lives. While medicine is a sophisticated scientific endeavor, it is also very much an art form, and every individual brings their own personality, commitments, and values to their practice. Hopefully this approach can ensure that the few instances when providers feel they must object will be taken seriously while enabling conscientious health care providers to take part in most interventions, thus mitigating conflicts and allowing all patients to receive both the medical treatments and the compassion that they deserve and our society to be served by medical professionals with a very strong moral compass and commitment to patient-centered care.

## NOTES

1. Shoni Davis, Vivian Schrader, and Marcia J. Belcheir, "Influencers of Ethical Beliefs and the Impact on Moral Distress and Conscientious Objection," *Nursing Ethics* 19 (2012): 738–49; Farr A. Curlin, Ryan E. Lawrence, Marshall H. Chin, and John D. Landos, "Religion, Conscience, and Controversial Clinical Practices," *New England Journal of Medicine* 356 (2007): 593–600; and Farr A. Curlin, Chinyere Nwodim, Jennifer L. Vance, Marshall H. Chin, and John D. Lantos, "To Die, to Sleep: US Physicians' Religious and Other Objections to Physician-Assisted Suicide, Terminal Sedation, and Withdrawal of Life," *American Journal of Hospice and Palliative Medicine* 25, no. 2 (2008): 112–20.

2. Jere Odell, Rahul Abhyankar, Amber Malcom, and Avril Rua, "Conscientious Objection in Health Professions: A Reader's Guide to the Ethical and Social Issues" (June 14, 2014), retrieved from https://scholarworks.iupui.edu/bitstream/handle/1805/4531/conscientiousobjectionscope.pdf?sequence=1andisAllowed=y.

3. When King Saul ordered the commanders of his army to execute all of the innocent Kohanim of the city of Nov (I Sam. 22:17), they refused to carry out the king's orders because there was no duty to obey the king if his order was sinful (see *Radak* there; *Sanhedrin* 49a, *Rashi* s.v. *sheheim darshu*). Prior to that, the first recorded instance of civil disobedience is that of the midwives, Shifra and Puah, whose fear of God motivated them to refuse to obey the immoral order of the Egyptian king to kill the Jewish baby boys (Ex. 1:17–21); see discussion in Jonathan Sacks, *Covenant & Conversation, a Weekly Reading of the Jewish Bible: Exodus* (New Milford, CT: Maggid, 2010), 21.

4. Margaret W. Beal and Joyce Capiello, "Professional Right of Conscience," *Journal of Midwifery and Women's Health* 53 (2008): 406–12.

5. *Roe v. Wade*, 410 US 113 (1973). The legal concept of "conscientious objection" dates back at least to the 1948 Universal Declaration of Human Rights. Article 18 states, "Everyone has the right to freedom of thought, conscience, and religion." Thaddeus Mason Pope, "Legal Briefing: Conscience Clauses and Conscientious Refusal," *Journal of Clinical Ethics* 21, no. 2 (2010): 163–80.

6. Pope, 163–80.

7. Christian Munthe, "Conscientious Refusal in Health Care: The Swedish Solution," *Journal of Medical Ethics* 43 (2017): 257–59; and Pope, "Legal Briefing," 163–80.

8. Daniel P. Sulmasy, "Tolerance, Professional Judgment, and the Discretionary Space of the Physician," *Cambridge Quarterly of Healthcare Ethics* 26 (2017): 18–31; and Daniel Weinstock, "Conscientious Refusal and Health Professionals: Does Religion Make a Difference," *Bioethics* 28, no. 1 (2014): 8–15.

9. Mark R. Wicclair, "Conscientious Objection in Medicine," *Bioethics* 14, no. 3 (2000): 207; Stephen Wear, Susan Lagaipa, and Gerald Logue, "Toleration of Moral Diversity and the Conscientious Refusal by Physicians to Withdraw Life-Sustaining Treatment," *Journal of Medicine and Philosophy* 19 (1994): 147–59; and H. Tristram Engelhardt, *The Foundations of Bioethics* (New York: Oxford University Press, 1986).

10. Daniel P. Sulmasy, "What Is Conscience and Why Is Respect for It So Important?" *Theoretical Medicine and Bioethics* 29, no. 3 (2008): 144.

11. Bernard M. Dickens and Rebecca J. Cook, "The Scope and Limits of Conscientious Objection," *International Journal of Gynecology and Obstetrics* 71, no. 1 (2000): 71–77.

12. Julie Cantor and Ken Baum, "The Limits of Conscientious Objection—May Pharmacists Refuse to Fill Prescriptions for Emergency Contraception?" *New England Journal of Medicine* 351, no. 19 (November 4, 2004): 2008–12.

13. Jason T. Eberl, "Conscientious Objection in Health Care," *Theoretical Medicine and Bioethics* 40 (2019): 483–86, https://doi.org/10.1007/s11017-019-09511-x.

14. Kimberley Brownlee, *Conscience and Conviction: The Case for Civil Disobedience* (Oxford: Oxford University Press, 2012), 128–39, 167–68, 171–72.

15. Bjørn K. Myskja and Morten Magelssen, "Conscientious Objection to Intentional Killing: An Argument for Toleration," *BMC Medical Ethics* 19, no. 82 (2018), https://doi.org/10.1186s12910-018-0323-0.

16. Cantor and Baum, "Limits of Conscientious Objection," 2008–12.

17. Mark R. Wicclair, "Conscientious Objection, Moral Integrity, and Professional Obligations," *Perspectives in Biology and Medicine* 62, no. 3 (2019): 543–59; Martin Benjamin, "Conscience," in *Encyclopedia of Bioethics*, ed. Warren T. Reich, 3rd ed. (New York: Simon and Schuster Macmillan, 2004), 514; James F. Childress, "Appeals to Conscience," *Ethics* 89, no. 4 (1979): 315–35; James F. Childress, "Conscience and Conscientious Actions in the Context of MCOs," *Kennedy Institute of Ethics Journal* 7, no. 4 (1997): 403–11; and Jeffrey Blustein, "Doing What the Patient Orders: Maintaining Integrity in the Doctor-Patient Relationship," *Bioethics* 7, no. 4 (1993): 289–314.

18. James F. Childress and Mark Siegler, "Metaphors and Models of Doctor-Patient Relationships: Their Implications for Autonomy," *Theoretical Medicine* 5, no. 1 (1984): 17–30; and Eva M. Norberg, Helge Skirbekk, and Morten Maggelson, "Conscientious Objection to Referrals for Abortion: Pragmatic Solution or Threat to Women's Rights?" *BMC Medical Ethics* 15, no. 15 (2014), https://doi.org/10.1186/1472-6939-15-15.

19. Wicclair, "Conscientious Objection, Moral Integrity"; Vicki D. Lachman, "Conscientious Objection in Nursing: Definition and Criteria for Acceptance," *MedSurg Nursing* 23,

no. 3 (2014): 196–98; and Lilia Susana Meltzer and Loucine Missak Huckabay, "Critical Care Nurses' Perceptions of Futile Care and Its Impact on Burnout," *American Journal of Critical Care* 13 (2004): 202–8.

20. Mary Neal and Sara Fovargue, "Is Conscientious Objection Incompatible with Healthcare Professionalism?" *New Bioethics* 25, no. 3 (2019): 221–35.

21. Charles D. Hepler, "Balancing Pharmacists' Conscientious Objections with Their Duty to Serve," *Journal of the American Pharmacists Association* 45, no. 4 (2005): 434.

22. For example, medical students and residents have successfully objected to performing educational procedures on corpses without their premortem consent as well as the use of animals in medical schools, and studies have shown that many medical students have felt pressured to act unethically, which hindered their ethical growth. Lisa K. Hicks, Yulia Lin, David W. Robertson, Deborah L. Robinson, and Sarah I. Woodrow, "Understanding the Clinical Dilemmas That Shape Medical Students' Ethical Development: Questionnaire Survey and Focus Group Study," *British Medical Journal* 322, no. 7288 (March 24, 2001): 709. On premortem consent, see Mark W. Fourre, "The Performance of Procedures on the Recently Deceased," *Academic Emergency Medicine* 9, no. 6 (2002): 595. On the use of animals in medical schools, see Susan Dodge, "Under Pressure from Students, Medical Schools Offer Alternatives to the Use of Live Animal Experiments," *Chronicle of Higher Education*, November 15, 1989, A41, A43.

23. Morten Magelssen, "When Should Conscientious Objection Be Accepted?" *Journal of Medical Ethics* 38 (2011): 18–21.

24. Neal and Fovargue, "Is Conscientious Objection Incompatible with Healthcare Professionalism?" 221–35.

25. Mark R. Wicclair, "Is Conscientious Objection Incompatible with a Physician's Professional Obligations?" *Theoretical Medicine and Bioethics* 29 (2008): 171–85. A related argument makes the point that just as medical professionals are sometimes free to refrain from offering services based on their personal interests or professional skills, they must also be allowed to refrain based on moral or religious objections. Aaron Ancell and Walter Sinnot-Armstrong, "How to Allow Conscientious Objection in Medicine While Protecting Patient Rights," *Cambridge Quarterly of Healthcare Ethics* 26, no. 1 (2017): 120–31.

26. Neal and Fovargue, "Is Conscientious Objection Incompatible with Healthcare Professionalism?" 221–35; Udo Schuklenk and Ricardo Smalling, "Why Medical Professionals Have No Moral Claim to Conscientious Objection Accommodation in Liberal Democracies," *Journal of Medical Ethics* 43, no. 4 (2017): 234–40; and Mark R. Wicclair, *Conscientious Objection in Health Care: An Ethical Analysis* (Cambridge: Cambridge University Press, 2011), xi. For discussion of some of the moral dilemmas this can lead to, see Tom L. Beauchamp and James F. Childress, *Principles of Biomedical Ethics*, 8th ed. (New York: Oxford University Press, 2019), 355.

27. Ronit Y. Stahl and Ezekiel J. Emanuel, "Physicians, Not Conscripts—Conscientious Objection in Health Care," *New England Journal of Medicine* 376, no. 14 (2017): 1380–85. Some have argued against conscientious objection in health care by pointing to a parallel to the military context, which is that those who object to participation are required by the military to engage in some form of alternative service and so, too, they argue, should

medical professionals who are unwilling to perform all of their duties. Eva LaFollette and Hugh LaFollette, "Private Conscience, Public Acts," *Journal of Medical Ethics* 33, no. 5 (2007): 249–54.

28. Julie D. Cantor, "Conscientious Objection Gone Awry—Restoring Selfless Professionalism in Medicine," *New England Journal of Medicine* 360 (April 9, 2009): 1484–85; and Julian Savulescu, "Conscientious Objection in Medicine," *British Medical Journal* 332, no. 7536 (February 4, 2006): 294. For these reasons, for example, in Sweden there is no right to conscientious objection. The Swedes argue that this is ethically correct since employers have the choice of reassigning employees on a case-by-case basis, and employees can choose not to take a job if they are uncomfortable with their duties. Munthe, "Conscientious Refusal in Health Care"; and Stahl and Emanuel, "Physicians, Not Conscripts."

29. Stahl and Emanuel; and Savulescu, "Conscientious Objection in Medicine," 294.

30. Savulescu, 294.

31. Savulescu, 294.

32. Wicclair, "Conscientious Objection, Moral Integrity," 543–59; and Cantor and Baum, "Limits of Conscientious Objection." For example, a California telephone survey found that refusals to fill emergency contraception were more common in rural areas. Olivia Sampson, Sandy K. Navarro, Amna Khan, Norman Hearst, Tina R. Raine, Marji Gold, Suellen Miller, and Heike Thiel de Bocanegra, "Barriers to Adolescents' Getting Emergency Contraception through Pharmacy Access in California: Differences by Language and Region," *Perspectives on Sexual and Reproductive Health* 41 (2009): 110–18. Studies have also shown that restrictions on abortion in some states render access to abortion extremely limited and sometimes insurmountable in some parts of the country. Wicclair, "Conscientious Objection, Moral Integrity," 543–59. Similarly, in all of Southern Italy, lawfully permitted abortions are not available anywhere since so few physicians are willing to perform them. Dickens and Cook, "Scope and Limits of Conscientious Objection." Furthermore, those who don't have health insurance, who rely on public or faith-based hospitals, and who have the fewest options—often racial and ethnic minorities—are also disproportionately the most negatively impacted by conscientious objection laws.

33. Savulescu, "Conscientious Objection in Medicine," 294; and Cantor, "Limits of Conscientious Objection," 2008–12. This includes racial, socioeconomic, and religious discrimination. This possibility is especially problematic since it is difficult to distinguish conscientious objection from objection from false motivations, such as cowardice or dislike. Lachman, "Conscientious Objection in Nursing," 196–98.

34. Lisa H. Harris, "Recognizing Conscience in Abortion Provision," *New England Journal of Medicine* 367 (September 13, 2012): 981–83.

35. Harris.

36. Neal and Fovargue, "Is Conscientious Objection Incompatible with Healthcare Professionalism?" 221–35; and Beal and Capiello, "Professional Right of Conscience," 406–12.

37. Neal and Fovargue, "Is Conscientious Objection Incompatible with Healthcare Professionalism?" 221–35; Beal and Capiello, "Professional Right of Conscience," 406–12; and Eberl, "Protecting Reasonable Conscientious Refusals in Health Care."

38. Lawrence Nelson, "Provider Conscientious Refusal of Abortion, Obstetrical

Emergencies, and Criminal Homicide Law," *American Journal of Bioethics* 18, no. 7 (2018): 43–50.

39. Anne Drapkin Lyerly, "Ethical Issues in Reproduction," in *Guidance for Healthcare Ethics Committees*, ed. D. Micah Hester and Toby Schonfeld (Cambridge: Cambridge University Press, 2012), 99; and Beal and Capiello, "Professional Right of Conscience," 406–12. See discussion in Beauchamp and Childress, *Principles of Biomedical Ethics*, 43–44.

40. Lyerly, "Ethical Issues in Reproduction"; and Beal and Capiello, "Professional Right of Conscience."

41. Roger Trigg, "Conscientious Objection and 'Effective Referral,'" *Cambridge Quarterly of Healthcare Ethics* 26, no. 1 (2017): 32–43; and Norberg et al., "Conscientious Objection to Referrals for Abortion."

42. Ancell and Sinnot-Armstrong, "How to Allow Conscientious Objection in Medicine"; and Savulescu, "Conscientious Objection in Medicine," 294.

43. *Torat Kohanim* 2:14.

44. *Pesachim* 22a; *Mo'ed Katan* 17a; and *Bava Metzia* 75b.

45. *Avodah Zarah* 6b.

46. *Avodah Zarah* 6b. See extensive discussion of this ruling in Rabbi Yair Hindin, "*Lifnei Iver*: When Best Practice Conflicts with Religious Practice," in *Sacred Training: A Halakhic Guidebook for Medical Students and Residents*, ed. Jerry Karp and Matthew Schaikewitz (New York: Ammud, 2018), 181–83.

47. Hindin, 181–83.

48. *Tosafot, Shabbat* 3a, s.v. *bava*; and Ritva and Ran, *Avodah Zarah* 6b, based on *Gittin* 61a.

49. *Avodah Zarah* 14a.

50. Mishnah, *Avodah Zarah* 4:9; Responsa *Binyan Tziyon* 1:15; Responsa *Mashiv Davar* 2:32 (he adds that this would be prohibited only if one causes the action to happen sooner than it would have; otherwise it is never prohibited to assist); and Responsa *Minchat Asher* 2:28, 30.

51. Responsa *Melamed LeHo'il* 1:34.

52. Ritva, *Gittin* 61a, s.v. *mashelet ishah*; Responsa *Mashiv Davar* 2:32; *Tzitz Eliezer* 19:33:9; *Shiurei Torah LeRofim* 4:246(2), 269; and Y. Schechter, *Kuntres Harofeh LeShevurei Lev: Psychotherapy in Halachah*, 72, 74.

53. *Iggerot Moshe*, YD 1:72 explaining *Shach*, YD 151:6 and *Dagul MeRevavah*, YD 151:6. See detailed discussions of this ruling in *Masorat Moshe*, 4:321–22; Hindin, "*Lifnei Iver*," 184–85; and Yitzchak Schechter, *Kuntres Harofeh LeShevurei Lev: Psychotherapy in Halachah* (New York: printed by the author, 2021), 67. See also *Yabia Omer* 9: OC108(190).

54. *Iggerot Moshe*, YD 1:72. Rabbi Feinstein argues that even those who disagree with his approach would agree in the case of permitting renting a hall to Jews who will use it for Jewishly inappropriate activities since the alternative is for them simply to rent another hall where they won't serve kosher food, so it would compound their transgression of Jewish law. Furthermore, Rabbi S. Z. Auerbach writes in Responsa *Minchat Shlomo* 1:35(1) that one may give food to a nonobservant Jew who will not cover their head or recite the required blessings since forcing them to do so could cause people to hate the Torah or religious Jews. This ruling is based on Rabbi A. Eiger's commentary on *Yoreh De'ah* 181:6 that since the Torah prohibits a man from shaving his face with a razor but doesn't prohibit a woman,

it would be better for a man who is going to shave his face with a razor anyway to have a woman do it for him, even though she is thus violating the prohibition of placing a stumbling block (or only the rabbinic prohibition of "assisting" since he can do it himself). Rabbi A. Eiger argues that when an action is prohibited by the Torah only due to placing a stumbling block in front of another, then it is better for a person to perform such an action since this way ultimately fewer sins will be committed. See also *Shiurei Torah LeRofim* 6:478, 597, which says that whenever one's actions will ultimately lead to long-term positive results, it is not considered a "stumbling block"; see also explanation of Rabbi A. Lichtenstein on this point in Hindin, "*Lifnei Iver*," 176.

55. For those who do not accept this approach, see Responsa *Minchat Shlomo* 3:103(4); Steinberg, *HaRefuah KeHalakhah* 2:380; and *Nishmat Avraham*, OC 656:1(3) (820–21 in 3rd ed.); see also Rosman, *Petichat HaIggeret*, 356. For those who do accept this approach, see Responsa *Maharit* 1:97; Responsa *Minchat Asher* 2:28–30 and vol. 4 (forthcoming).

56. Bryant Carlson, Nicole Simopolous, Elizabeth R. Goy, Ann Jackson, and Linda Ganzini, "Oregon Hospice Chaplains' Experiences with Patients Requesting Physician-Assisted Suicide," *Journal of Palliative Medicine* 8, no. 6 (2005): 1165; and Linda Ganzini and Steven K. Dobscha, "If It Isn't Depression . . . ," *Journal of Palliative Medicine* 6, no. 6 (2003): 927–30.

57. Dale A. Matthews, Anthony L. Suchman, and William T. Branch Jr., "Making 'Connexions': Enhancing the Therapeutic Potential of Patient-Clinician Relationships," *Annals of Internal Medicine* 118, no. 12 (1993): 973–77.

58. Lisa Rosenbaum, "Perilous Politics—Morbidity and Mortality in the Post-Roe Era," *New England Journal of Medicine* 381 (2019): 893–95; and David A. Grimes, Janie Benson, Susheela Singh, Mariana Romero, Bela Ganatra, Friday E. Okonofua, and Iqbal H. Shah, "Unsafe Abortion: The Preventable Pandemic," *Lancet* 368 (2006): 1908–19.

59. *Nishmat Avraham* 3;5 (159 in 3rd ed.); see also Hindin, "*Lifnei Iver*," 179.

60. Responsa *Minchat Asher*, vol. 4 (forthcoming); see also Hindin, "*Lifnei Iver*," 186. It is important to point out that there is also room for leniency when there is a likelihood that even if facilitated, the sin will not end up occurring. Responsa *Shevet HaLevi*, YD 62 based on *Shulchan Arukh*, YD 151:1.

61. Responsa *Minchat Asher*, vol. 4 (forthcoming) and 2:30(6). On the other hand, Rabbi Zilberstein writes that when such a committee allows an abortion that would not be permitted by Jewish law, an observant Jew must either excuse themselves from that committee or clearly protest the decision. *Shiurei Torah LeRofim* 6:464, 559.

62. *Nishmat Avraham*, YD 339:4(7) (510 in 3rd ed.). Rabbi M. Feinstein also explains why this would be permitted in many scenarios, but he suggests removing oneself from the situation if possible and prohibits it in certain scenarios (*Iggerot Moshe*, YD 4:54).

63. *Nishmat Avraham*, YD 339:1(4) (499 in 3rd ed.).

64. Responsa *Minchat Asher* (forthcoming; see quotation "Becoming a Physician: When Secular Law and Values Clash with Halacha," https://e8b7a5f9-e27e-4732-8c9b-1f83787ae640.filesusr.com/ugd/9c4394_7c5cdd45e1774f0c96fdbb00a3552fc9.pdf); *Tzitz Eliezer* 19:33(1). On the other hand, Rabbi Moshe Feinstein is quoted as ruling that it is forbidden to serve as an anesthesiologist for an abortion procedure (*Masorat Moshe*, 4:428).

65. Y. Schechter, *Kuntres Harofeh LeShevurei Lev: Psychotherapy in Halachah*, 59, in the name of Rabbi Dovid Cohen (see extensive analysis of the topic there).

66. Some argue that a health care provider should not impose their own religious commitments onto specific patients if doing so is likely to turn that patient off from seeking essential health care. Rabbi N. Bar-Ilan, quoted in Hoffman, *"Dilemot vekonfliktim hilkhati'im umusari'im bahem nitkalim psichologim dati'im,"* November 11, 2008, https://www.hebpsy.net/articles.asp?id=1896), particularly because health care providers engaging in their professional duties does not imply formal religious approval of their patients' actions and should therefore not be seen as "assisting" their sin. Rabbi S. Rappaport, https://www.hebpsy.net/articles.asp?id=1896, November 11, 2008. I thank Rabbi M. Torczyner for pointing these two sources out to me. On the importance of ensuring that there are religious doctors, see *Chelkat Yaakov*, YD 190(1).

# CHAPTER EIGHT

# Self-Care in Challenging Times

Having examined the duties and obligations of health care providers, it is crucial to begin to conclude by asking how far health care providers can realistically be expected to go on behalf of their patients. Self-care and burnout are important topics in health care. For example, during the COVID-19 pandemic, severe psychological distress and mental health struggles have been noticed among the general population as well as frontline health care providers in particular, including increased symptoms of panic disorder, anxiety, exhaustion, depression, posttraumatic stress, and suicide.[1] As a result, many have left the field of medicine or retired early.[2] In this chapter I thoroughly examine the expectations of health care providers and the extent of their duties, including some of the lessons and insights that are being learned from the COVID-19 pandemic, to suggest an innovative way of framing requirements of self-care and applying classical Jewish sources to this issue.

Many people enter the health care profession out of a profound desire to help others in need.[3] They frequently take on responsibility and burdens to care for others. Sometimes, whether due to chronic illness, severe pain, mental illness, contagious disease, or numerous other factors, patient demands can test the limits of a health care provider's skills and patience. Nevertheless, some seem to claim that there are no limits to health care providers' duties. For example, in a popular contemporary rendition of the Hippocratic oath, a health care provider pledges to "treat without exception all who seek my ministrations."[4] So, too, at the beginning of this century, the American Medical Association adopted a "Social Contract with Humanity," in which it commits the community of physicians to "apply our knowledge and skills when needed, though doing so may put us at risk."[5] Some Jewish bioethicists have suggested that we should not only ask about the minimal standards of medicine but should also seek to understand maximal standards and a health care provider's "ceaseless responsibility."[6]

Along these lines, a leading rabbinic scholar of the past generation, Rabbi Yaakov Yisrael Kanievsky (who was known as "the Steipler Gaon"), was once asked by someone if he should become a rabbi in a city with very few other observant Jews or if he should become a doctor and live wherever he chose. Rabbi Kanievsky responded that it would be much better for him to become a rabbi rather than a doctor since it is extremely difficult to truly fulfill all of the obligations Jewish law expects of doctors, which include the requirement to do everything humanly possible to save a patient's life without any concern for one's personal loss of money or time.[7] Some rabbinic thinkers have argued that health care professionals may never even keep patients waiting unnecessarily or else they would violate the Torah's prohibition of *inui hadin* (delaying a judgment).[8] Indeed, even during the most intense periods of the COVID-19 pandemic, some rabbinic authorities ruled that health care professionals were required to continue working in hospitals and as first responders even if they were afraid to care for contagious COVID patients.[9]

But Judaism also recognizes a duty to care for oneself and maintain one's own physical and mental well-being.[10] How can that demand be balanced with the duty to care for others? Are there limits to the extent that one is expected to go to on behalf of a patient? Must one spend all their surplus time and income for this cause or live an especially modest lifestyle in order to be able to achieve these ends? Personal danger, physical or emotional exhaustion, and difficult or noncompliant patients can be challenging aspects of contemporary health care. May one never take a break or ever say "no" to any patient's request for treatment?

This chapter examines the basis for the duty to provide health care and some potential limitations to that duty from the perspective of classical Jewish sources and some contemporary rabbinic thinkers. The chapter then compares and contrasts these Jewish sources with parallel discussions in the general bioethics literature in order to suggest a focused and rigorous understanding that arises out of applying classical interpretations of specific biblical verses to this issue. It then suggests a unique approach, based on the rabbinic laws of charity, that can help articulate an optimal level of obligation.


## THE BASIS AND IMPORTANCE OF A HEALTH CARE PROVIDER'S DUTY TO TREAT

By analyzing the very foundation of the basis for a health care provider's responsibilities, we can begin to formulate an approach to this issue. Both classical

Jewish thought and contemporary bioethical literate examine this issue in great detail and have some important similarities as well as differences.

## A Jewish Approach

The Torah considers providing health care to be a "mitzvah," as is visiting and supporting the sick, and regards practicing medicine as an act of imitating God's ways.[11] Judaism does not require one to become a health care professional, but as one trains and develops lifesaving skills, a person becomes required to use those skills whenever the need arises.[12] Not only is providing health care thus a positive duty, but the Torah also prohibits a person from "standing idly by" when there is something they can do to help another person in need of lifesaving assistance.[13] The rabbis criticized those who have the ability to care for the sick but do not do so, going so far as to regard health care professionals who do not treat people in need as being guilty of murder.[14]

## A Bioethics Approach

The bioethical literature also includes discussions on the source of a health care professional's duty to provide care. Some claim a "common morality," mandating that all people are expected to help others who are in need.[15] As with Jewish values, secular bioethicists also maintain that this duty to provide care becomes especially true once one develops the necessary training and skills and is in a position to help others, even if that means taking some risks to do so.[16] Another basis for the duty to provide care, known as "implied consent" or "express consent," is the argument that by accepting a job as a health care provider, one is implicitly consenting to the risks and expectations associated with that field along with its obligations.[17] Indeed, many point to the professional oaths and codes that many health care providers take, most of which require significant risk and self-sacrifice on behalf of one's patients.[18]

One of the most-cited sources in the bioethics literature for a health care provider's obligation to go out of their way for others is the concept of "reciprocity," which is itself intertwined with the notion of a "social contract" inherent in professional service.[19] This line of reasoning points out that health care providers receive numerous benefits from society, such as government/taxpayer subsidized education and training, prestige, and self-regulation/autonomy, which affords them greater trust and access to medicine, protective measures, treatments, and so on as well as state licensure that affords them exclusivity and opportunities for higher salaries. In light of these advantages, the argument is that it is reasonable to expect the recipients of these benefits (most health care providers) to provide a public service and even to put themselves at more risk than the average person.[20] Some further argue that this special training and status, coupled with patients' vulnerability (especially those who are hospitalized and at the mercy of the staff[21]), creates a duty for health care providers to put any patient's needs and welfare above their own self-interests.[22]

Encouragement for individuals to take on the roles and duties of health care providers, both from Jewish sources and bioethics literature, is evident. However, not all health care professionals are members of specific professional organizations or take oaths (which are generally not binding anyway), nor does every health care provider receive the same amount of benefit from society. Still, underlying this discussion is a basic assumption about duty and morality—that is, that all people are expected to contribute to other people's welfare, which is a key principle in both Judaism and bioethics known as beneficence.

## BENEFICENCE

The goal and justification for health care is not just to avoid causing harm but includes the positive duty to take steps that aim to provide benefit to patients.[23] In bioethics, this principle is known as "beneficence," or doing good. It is often traced directly to the Torah's commandment to love one's neighbor as oneself and has played a central role in many ethical theories throughout history.[24] The rabbis codified this principle as a matter of Jewish law and "the great principle of the Torah," and it is a basis in Jewish law for the requirement to provide health care (see note 24 and extensive discussion in chapter 6).[25] Therefore, many argue that Judaism demands a higher level of beneficence than secular bioethics, or prioritizes it higher, because actively doing good for others is not just praiseworthy or seen as appropriate or going "above and beyond" but is an ethical obligation in Judaism.[26]

Furthermore, Jewish law requires that one provide "beneficence" to all, not just one's relatives or patients.[27] By contrast, within the general bioethics liter-ature, most agree that one owes basic duties of beneficence only toward those with whom they are in a relationship, such as family members or patients (this is known as "specific beneficence").[28] However, debate is found within the bioethics literature as to whether any "general" expectations of beneficence are owed equally to all. Some have argued that health care providers do have an obligation of "general beneficence" based on "the mere fact that there are other human beings in the world whose condition we can make better."[29] But many other bioethicists are concerned that such a "general" requirement is impractical and diverts necessary attention away from those specific individuals to whom a health care provider owes clear responsibilities.[30] One may choose to go over and above one's basic obligations but cannot be expected to do so for all people since one has different levels of obligations for different people (i.e., family members, their own patients, strangers).[31] Some bioethicists maintain that a moral obligation of general beneficence does not exist but rather it is a moral ideal.[32] Moreover, some limit this beneficence to the promotion of patient health but not their overall well-being.[33] Consensus can be found in the bioethics literature that, at a minimum, when one is well positioned and capable of offering assistance to another person, the moral expectation of beneficence would at least include accepting some risks/burdens to do so, although not necessarily significant risks, costs, or burdens (the precise level of these risks is difficult to define).[34]

Similarly, although Jewish law regards "general beneficence" as an obligation for an individual's overall well-being, not just their health, Jewish law agrees that there are limits as to how far one must endanger themselves for others. For example, Jewish law does not expect lay people to place themselves at significant risk to save others, but it obligates health care professionals to put themselves at greater risk, even to care for patients with a contagious illness.[35] Jewish law regards these risks inherent for a medical professional as a necessary aspect of normal societal function and their professional responsibilities, just as society may expect soldiers to risk their lives for their country during a war.[36] Some secular bioethicists express a concern that assuming such risks by treating a highly contagious illness could lead to a shortage of medical professionals, thus endangering the public, which is what has happened during the COVID-19 pandemic in some places.[37] The COVID-19 pandemic also has raised concerns related to health care professionals transmitting the disease to their family members, especially those who are elderly, immunocompromised, or have chronic medical conditions.[38] Rabbinic authorities have expressed similar caution but emphasize communal responsibilities by contending that medical professionals must proactively endanger themselves by treating patients with contagious illness for the sake of public safety in order to prevent a mass outbreak.[39] However, this does not mean that Jewish law requires one to engage in any level of severe risk without limitation.

## LIMITS

The rabbis of the Talmud recognized that some limits to the responsibilities and expectations of health care professionals are necessary or no one would go into the profession or be able to maintain that lifestyle.[40] Although some rabbinic authorities argue that a doctor must be available at all times, most recognize that doctors need to take breaks or have times when they are not on call (assuming others are available who can care for dangerously ill patients or respond to urgent needs).[41] Indeed, Jewish law stipulates that one may not take on additional jobs outside of their normal professional obligations if these responsibilities could exhaust them or render them unable to fulfill their primary obligations.[42] This professional limitation suggests that it can sometimes be inappropriate to go above and beyond for patients if it will decrease the quality of care one is able to provide for other patients.[43] Furthermore, if a health care professional takes on too many patients or does not take breaks, they are more likely to make medical errors, which Jewish law considers an irresponsible outcome and therefore holds health care professionals liable for even inadvertent mistakes.[44] A general restriction on overextending oneself can thus be seen, which is highlighted for health care professionals since the stakes of their professional obligations and potential for error are so high.

Similarly, the general contemporary practice of medicine includes very extensive support for limits on health care providers' duties. For example, if a patient fails to adhere to their medical regimen, behaves inappropriately, does not pay their bills, and so on, clinicians may sometimes "fire" their patients as long as they provide reasonable notice and cause (when done without reasonable notice or justification, this is known as "patient abandonment"[45]). A health care provider can also choose not to provide a certain procedure if it is outside of their competence, if it is determined to be medically futile, or if they have a conscience-based objection.[46]

However, some bioethicists have proposed broader philosophical grounds to support limiting a health care provider's duties in various circumstances. One perspective within the bioethics literature emphasizes the fact that, in addition to duties toward others, one also has a responsibility to care for oneself and maintain one's own well-being.[47] At one time, medical education focused primarily on inculcating a strong work ethic, professionalism, stamina, and self-sacrifice, but today the focus has moved toward developing compassion, empathy, and self-care and recognizing that being overworked can drain one's compassion and motivation and lead to burnout, errors, and harm to patients.[48] Furthermore, an inexhaustible amount of suffering occurs in the world, and for health care providers to be expected to alleviate all of it would be psychologically debilitating. Recognizing human finite capacities by limiting beneficence and expectations of duty is thus essential for health care providers to maintain their ability to function effectively over the course of their careers.[49]

Excessively high expectations for health care providers to risk their own well-being for the sake of others could also compromise public welfare. For example, if too many providers were to become ill themselves and thus unable to care for others, that could lead to a shortage of health care professionals, which could result in increased danger to everyone in society.[50] Some bioethicists express concerns similar to those raised by the rabbis of the Talmud, maintaining that unreasonably high expectations to endanger oneself for patients could result in disincentives to enter the health care profession, which would exacerbate shortages and be detrimental to public health, especially during pandemics.[51]

Parallels between Jewish and bioethics concerns are clear, as are some distinctions. For example, both suggest a desire to prevent disincentives from entering the health care profession and a recognition that a health care professional must engage in good self-care in order to be able to practice medicine optimally and avoid harm to self and patients. The Jewish perspective that we have examined seems to be slightly more demanding, using stronger language of "obligation" and stressing communal concerns above individual needs. This obligation, which may give rise to unique limitations on health care providers' duties, derives from specific sources.

## RETURNING LOST OBJECTS

Although attempting to heal the sick is a commandment of the Torah, some debate is found in rabbinic literature as to which verse in the Torah commands it. One answer is that the verse "Do not stand idly by . . . " obligates anyone who can help a patient who is enduring tremendous suffering or has a very serious illness to do whatever they can do for that individual.[52] However, if the patient's illness is certainly not life threatening, the requirement to attempt to help someone regain their health is based on the verse that requires returning lost objects, "You shall give it back" (i.e., help to return their health to them), as discussed in chapter 3 of this book.[53]

Although basing health care on this commandment implies very demanding expectations of health care providers because one must show concern for returning anyone's lost object anytime they encounter it, there is also much more flexibility since Jewish law does not always require returning every lost object.[54] This verse does not require going to every extent possible or to suffer significant self-sacrifice or loss in order to do so.[55] For example, the Torah does not require enduring significant financial or personal loss in order to return a lost object, and neither, therefore, is one required to support such a patient, although doing so would certainly be considered meritorious.[56] This obligation does not require going further for others than one goes for themselves to recover lost objects, and it does not expect a total abnegation of the self or caring for others more than one cares for oneself.[57]

Although the verse requiring the return of lost objects is applied to health care, it might not apply in all situations. For example, the Talmud rules that "even a prominent person must visit a lowly person who is sick," requiring one to support even those they might perceive as being beneath their status.[58] However, included in the laws of returning lost objects, a distinguished person for whom it would be beneath their dignity to have to return the object is exempt from the requirement.[59] The requirements of visiting and supporting the sick thus go beyond those of returning lost objects.[60] Deriving clear parallels to all modern health care situations from the specific laws of returning lost objects is thus sometimes challenging. Identifying a more specific approach to help clarify the extent of a health care provider's duty is thus crucial.

## THE ONE-FIFTH RULE

A limitation on how far one is required to go to fulfill Jewish law and the parameters of its application can be expounded from a different Jewish legal category based on a unique interpretation of another verse. Regarding the verse in the Torah, "Everything that you give me I will tithe to You" (Gen. 28:22), the rabbis decreed that "when one dispenses their money to charity, they should not dispense more than one-fifth."[61] The reason for this limitation is that the Torah does not want one to spend all their money on one mitzvah since that would leave them destitute and unable to perform other meritorious acts.[62] Rather, one is expected to carefully ration the way they distribute their resources, despite any of the Torah's obligations.[63] The rabbis determined that one-fifth of one's wealth is the maximum that one may spend on fulfilling the requirements of any given positive commandment.[64]

Some later rabbinic authorities have applied this principle to areas beyond financial concerns in a novel fashion. They argue that just as one is not required to spend a large sum to fulfill a commandment, neither are they expected to become physically ill in order to do so because a person's financial well-being should not be more important to them than their physical well-being.[65] Since most people would be willing to spend much more than a fifth of their financial resources to avoid severe pain and suffering, some rabbinic authorities argue that enduring tremendous physical pain or emotional suffering or giving a large amount of one's time would be tantamount to spending more than a fifth of one's resources and is thus not required.[66] This approach therefore becomes a strong basis for limiting the extent to which heroic endeavors are taken in order to fulfill a positive commandment such as providing health care.

When it comes to saving a life, the amount of time, energy, or money that should be expended to do so has no limit. Many rabbinic authorities do indeed maintain that one must spend all they have to save a life, while others—including many contemporary rabbinic authorities—rule that one need not spend more than one-fifth of their assets even to save another's life.[67] This ruling recognizes that the obligation to save a life is shared by the entire community in order to protect the general public's financial viability.[68]

Similarly, Jewish values recognize a public obligation to provide health care for all (see chapter 3).[69] This public duty itself serves as a critical limitation on the duty of any particular health care provider because when the public does not provide sufficient human and medical resources to respond to the health care needs of the public, the duty of any particular health care provider is limited as well. Everyone in a society is expected to do their part by contributing to communal needs, but no individual can be required to spend everything they have in order to do it all on their own.[70]

While Jewish law expects people to endure some discomfort, pain, and suffering to fulfill commandments, how far these expectations go is limited (although people may sometimes choose to go above and beyond minimal expectations in certain circumstances[71]), and the one-fifth rule helps to frame and quantify these limits.[72] To expect a health care provider to be available at all times and do everything they can on behalf of any patient in need could drain all of a person's emotional and financial resources and jeopardize others to whom they owe responsibility, thus costing them more than one-fifth of their wealth. While quantifying emotional suffering is difficult, this approach helps to justify limitations and provide general guidelines and validation for the need to limit the extent of a health care provider's duties.

There are many ways individuals may be able to apply the one-fifth rule to different areas of their lives. During the COVID-19 pandemic, health care workers have experienced significant stress, burnout, and risks to their mental health, including mood and sleep disturbances.[73] One of the suggestions for coping with these problems is to promote flexibility and work-life integration for health care workers.[74] I would therefore suggest that—other than during periods of extreme crisis when one may need to work especially abnormal hours, such as adjusting to a "new normal" during a pandemic—they calculate their normal work schedule and be careful not to exceed that norm by more than 20 percent. Thus, if one normally works fifty hours per week, they should make sure not to begin working more than sixty hours per week on a regular basis. Similarly, if one normally takes fourteen days of vacation, they should not reduce that by more than 20 percent and still take at least eleven days of vacation that year.

## CONCLUSION

Many health care providers have been conditioned not to consider their own safety or well-being when caring for their patients. However, caring for oneself and applying limits to a health care provider's duties are not only vital but also philosophically and ethically defensible. Although the two approaches examined begin with very different foundations and assumptions—bioethics is often based primarily on philosophy and logic, while Jewish approaches tend to be based on interpretations of specific biblical verses and Talmudic tradition—they both come to many very similar conclusions. Both rabbinic and bioethics thinkers have expressed high expectations of health care providers as well as justifications for limiting those expectations when necessary. Both recognize that excessive demands may prevent people from entering the field, and both recognize that at times going above and beyond for one's patients is praiseworthy. Judaism seems to have slightly higher expectations of health care providers than many secular bioethicists (e.g., using the language of general obligation, limiting the possibility of even taking breaks, and regarding health care providers who do not provide care to be guilty of murder) but also offers very specific exemptions. The Jewish approaches examined also seem more focused on communal responsibilities than individual roles.

Within both traditions, even as limits on the duties of health care providers are set, the societal importance of the role of health care providers to care for the sick is maintained. The perspectives examined do not see health care providers merely as mechanics of the body but as individuals who have taken on themselves social and even divine expectations of responsibility to go out of their way for others. Both bioethics and the Jewish tradition demand that one who undergoes the training to care for people's health takes on an obligation to do so that cannot be taken lightly. Yet both perspectives recognize that human capabilities are limited and that a person cannot be expected to extend themselves unreasonably.[75] It turns out that central to an ethic of responsibility is responsibility to oneself.

Although setting very high expectations can encourage people to strive to live up to them, if the expectations are too demanding, many will become disillusioned and less likely to carry out even minimal moral duties.[76] Determining the right balance is thus crucial. The one-fifth rule can help establish an optimal level of obligation as it demands real self-sacrifice but also sets a clear and definite limit while granting subjective case-by-case calibration. As health care providers navigate the demands and struggles of providing care at all times, especially during a crisis, approaches such as this can help set proper limits and promote care provider well-being and longevity.

# NOTES

1. See the sources and research cited in Steven Pirutinsky, Aaron D. Cherniak, and David H. Rosmarin, "COVID-19, Mental Health, and Religious Coping among American Orthodox Jews," *Journal of Religion and Health* 59 (2020): 2288–2301, https://doi.org/10.1007/s10943-020-01070-z; and Agata Benfante, Marialaura Di Tella, Romeo Annunziata, and Lorys Castelli, "Traumatic Stress in Healthcare Workers during COVID-19 Pandemic: A Review of the Immediate Impact," *Frontiers in Psychology* 11 (October 2020), https://doi.org/10.3389/fpsyg.2020.569935.

2. Jordan Kisner, "What the Chaos in Hospitals Is Doing to Doctors," *Atlantic*, December 8, 2020, https://www.theatlantic.com/magazine/archive/2021/01/covid-ethics-committee/617261/.

3. Moheem Masumali Halari, Chidambra Dhariwal Halari, Olukayode Ahmed Busari, and Christopher James Watterson, "Motivational Factors for Aspiring Doctors," *American Scientific Research Journal for Engineering, Technology and Sciences* 19, no. 1 (2016): 103–12.

4. Value of Life Committee, "1995 Restatement of the Oath of Hippocrates," National Catholic Bioethics Center.

5. American Medical Association, "Declaration of Professional Responsibility: Medicine's Social Contract with Humanity," *Missouri Medicine* 99, no. 5 (2002): 195. One of the strongest statements of physician duty in the modern era appeared in the 1847 Code of Medical Ethics of the AMA: "When pestilence prevails, it is their [physician's] duty to face the danger, and to continue their labours for the alleviation of the suffering, even at the jeopardy of their own lives." See Tom L. Beauchamp and James F. Childress, *Principles of Biomedical Ethics*, 8th ed. (New York: Oxford University Press, 2019), 49.

6. Laurie Zoloth, *Second Texts/Second Opinions: Essays toward a Jewish Bioethics* (Oxford: Oxford University Press, 2022), chap. 6.

7. *Kreina DeIgrata* 1:201; and *Shiurei Torah LeRofim*, 2, 394–95.

8. Maharsham 2:210, cited in *Nishmat Avraham*, YD 336:1(5) (470 in 3rd ed.); Rabbi Zilberstein points out that a doctor may not take a break if not responding immediately could endanger someone's life, based on Rabbi Shimon ben Gamliel's concern in *Semachot* 8:8, and Nachum Ish Gamzu in *Ta'anit* 21a, that he was being punished for not answering rabbinic questions immediately (*Shiurei Torah LeRofim* 1:16, 200–201). Based on this, Rabbi Zilberstein argues that the reason no blessing is made by a doctor on fulfilling the commandment to heal is because it would be inappropriate to pause to pray, even momentarily, while a patient is waiting in pain, similar to God's rebuke of Moses for stopping to pray while the Jews were fleeing Egypt (Ex. 14:15, *Shemot Rabbah* 21:8).

9. Rabbi S. Kamenetsky, quoted in Kleinman, *Kovetz Halakhot, LiTekufat Choli Korona*, p. 365. Responsa *Shevet HaLevi* 8:251(7) ruled similarly based on the precedent of a similar ruling of Rabbi A. Eiger during the cholera outbreak one hundred years earlier. All of this assumes health care professionals take appropriate personal protective measures. See further discussion later in this chapter.

10. See discussion in Benjamin Freedman, *Duty and Healing: Foundations of a Jewish Bioethic* (New York: Routledge, 1999), 142–47, 176, 181, based on Ramchal, *Derekh Hashem* 1:4(7) and the laws of *shomrim*, such as *Shulchan Arukh*, CM 121, 290–91.

11. On providing health care as a "mitzvah," see *Shulchan Arukh*, YD 336:1. In fact, some have argued that practicing medicine is such an important profession that while one is practicing this profession, they are engaged in the fulfillment of a mitzvah, which cannot be said of almost any other profession. *Encyclopedia Hilkhatit Refu'it* 7, 180; see similar perspective in Rabbi Bakshi Doron, *Binyan Av: Refuah BeHalakhah*, 27–30, 206. Indeed, it is reported that Rabbi S. Salant told doctors who would study Torah in the mornings before going to work that they were needed more in the hospital and should go there right away instead of setting time to study Torah in the mornings, and that Rabbi Y. C. Zonnenfeld once told a doctor not to join communal activist gatherings because the best use of his time was to be in the hospital for his patients as much as possible; see *Shiurei Torah LeRofim* 6:393(4), 294–95. On visiting and supporting the sick, see *Shulchan Arukh*, YD 335:1. The Torah refers to God as a healer (Ex. 15:26). Based on this some argue that practicing medicine can be seen as a "calling." See David Novak, *The Sanctity of Human Life* (Washington, DC: Georgetown University Press, 2007), 101–2.

12. *Iggerot Moshe*, YD 2:151; *Shiurei Torah LeRofim* 6:312, 44.

13. Lev. 19:16. See *Tosafot HaRosh, Berakhot* 60a, s.v. *mikan shenitna.*

14. Rashi in *Kiddushin* 82a comments that the rabbinic saying that "the best of doctors go to hell" refers to one who can treat a patient but does not do so. See also *Shulchan Arukh*, YD 336:1.

15. Heidi Malm, Thomas May, Leslie P. Francis, Saad B. Omer, Daniel A. Salmon, and Robert Hood, "Ethics, Pandemics, and the Duty to Treat," *American Journal of Bioethics* 8, no. 8 (2008): 4–19; and Chalmers C. Clark, "In Harm's Way: AMA Physicians and the Duty to Treat," *Journal of Medicine and Philosophy* 30, no. 1 (2005): 82.

16. Malm et al., "Ethics, Pandemics, and the Duty to Treat," 4–19; and Clark, "In Harm's Way," 82.

17. Malm et al., "Ethics, Pandemics, and the Duty to Treat," 4–19; and Clark, "In Harm's Way," 82.

18. Malm et al., "Ethics, Pandemics, and the Duty to Treat," 4–19; Clark, "In Harm's Way," 82; and Linda Twardowski, Twila McInnis, Carleton C. Cappuccino, James McDonald, and Jason Rhodes, "Professional Responsibilities for Treatment of Patients with Ebola: Can a Healthcare Provider Refuse to Treat a Patient with Ebola?" *Rhode Island Medical Journal*, 97, no. 10 (2014): 63.

19. Malm et al., "Ethics, Pandemics, and the Duty to Treat," 9–10; Sandra J. Carnahan, "Concierge Medicine: Legal and Ethical Issues," *Journal of Law, Medicine and Ethics* 35, no. 1 (2007): 213; Martin Donohoe, "Luxury Primary Care, Academic Medical Centers, and

the Erosion of Science and Professional Ethics," *Journal of General Internal Medicine* 19, no. 1 (2004): 90–94; and Clark, "In Harm's Way," 82.

20. Malm et al., "Ethics, Pandemics, and the Duty to Treat," 9–10. Similarly, some thinkers argue that there is a moral right to government-funded health care based on this concept of reciprocity since society invests so much in medical education, biomedical research, and the medical system; see Beauchamp and Childress, *Principles of Biomedical Ethics*, 291.

21. Micah Johnson, "Do Physicians Have an Ethical Duty to Repair Relationships with So-Called 'Difficult' Patients?" *AMA Journal of Ethics* 19, no. 4 (2017): 325–26.

22. William Martinez and Thomas H. Gallagher, "Ethical Concierge Medicine?" *Virtual Mentor, American Medical Association Journal of Ethics* 15, no. 7 (2013): 577; Bernard Lo, "Retainer Medicine: Why Not for All?" *Annals of Internal Medicine* 155, no. 9 (2011): 641–42; and Richard L. Creuss and Sylvia R. Creuss, "Teaching Medicine as a Profession in the Service of Healing," *Academic Medicine* 72 (1997): 941–52.

23. Beauchamp and Childress, *Principles of Biomedical Ethics*, 217; *Encyclopedia of Bioethics*, 4th ed. (Macmillan Reference, 2014), 311.

24. Lev. 19:18. Ramban, *Torat HaAdam Sha'ar HaSakanah*, s.v. *aval rabbeinu*. The principles of beneficence and nonmaleficence can also find support in Psalm 34:14: "Turn from evil and do good." See also Beauchamp and Childress, *Principles of Biomedical Ethics*, 218.

25. *Sifra, Kedoshim* 2:4(12); *Shabbat* 31a.

26. On a higher level of beneficence than secular bioethics, see A. Steinberg, *Encyclopedia of Jewish Medical Ethics*, vol. 3 (Jerusalem: Feldheim, 2003), 386. Judaism includes many more commandments than "love your neighbor as yourself," such as specific requirements like honoring elders (Lev. 19:32) and caring for orphans and widows (Ex. 22:21–23). Indeed, in Jewish law, one can even be punished not just for damaging another but for not going out of their way to help them (see *Encyclopedia Hilkhatit Refu'it*, 7, 890).

27. Rambam, *Hilkhot De'ot* 6:3; and Rabbi P. Eliyahu, *Sefer HaBrit* 2:13.

28. J. Paul Kelleher, "Beneficence, Justice and Health Care," *Kennedy Institute of Ethics Journal* 24, no. 1 (2014): 31; and Beauchamp and Childress, *Principles of Biomedical Ethics*, 219–21.

29. William D. Ross, *The Right and the Good* (Oxford: Clarendon Press, 1930), 21.

30. Beauchamp and Childress, *Principles of Biomedical Ethics*, 220.

31. Beauchamp and Childress, 220.

32. Kelleher, "Beneficence, Justice and Health Care," 30. This perspective maintains that an obligation can arise only when one has a specific claim to receive beneficence from one with whom they are in a professional or familial relationship.

33. Kelleher, 45.

34. Beauchamp and Childress, *Principles of Biomedical Ethics*, 219–22.

35. On lay people, see *She'elot UTeshuvot HaRadvaz* 218 and 3:627; *Shulchan Arukh*, CM 426:1, *Sma* 2 and *Arukh HaShulchan* 4; and *Mishnah Berurah* 328:9. On health care professionals, see *Magen Avraham*, OC 574:6; *Tzitz Eliezer* 8:15(10:13) and 9:17; *Kuntres Refuah BeShabbat* 5:4–8; Responsa *Shevet HaLevi* 8:251(7); *Shiurei Torah LeRofim* 1:46; *Nishmat Avraham*, CM 426:2(4), 235 in 3rd ed.; and *HaRefuah KeHalakha* 8:1(9), 14. Rabbi A. Weiss also rules that a surgeon who is afraid of performing surgery on a patient with a contagious illness is nevertheless required to perform that surgery. Responsa *Minchat Asher* 3:121(2). Community members may continue

to visit patients with a contagious illness if they take all appropriate precautions. *Chazon Ovadia, Aveilut* 1, 14–15; *Tzitz Eliezer* 17:5(11); *HaRefuah KeHalakhah* 4:3, 2(6), 155; *Minchat Asher, Bereishit* 30 (7); Responsa *Minchat Asher* 3:122; and *Minchat Asher–Magefat HaKorona*, 11(3).

36. *Tzitz Eliezer* 9:17; *Kuntres Refuah BeShabbat* 5:7–9; and Responsa *Minchat Asher* 3:121(2). See discussion in Dovid Lichtenstein, *Headlines 2: Halachic Debates of Current Events* (New York: Oxford University Press, 2017), 274–78.

37. Marta Paterlini, "On the Front Lines of Coronavirus: The Italian Response to Covid-19," *BMJ* 368 (March 16, 2020), https://doi.org/10.1136/bmj.m1065. Similarly, R. Asher Weiss ruled that a first responder whose spouse is in a high-risk category should not engage in medical care for contagious patients so as not to endanger their spouse (*Minchat Asher–Magefat HaKorona*, 15).

38. James G. Adams and Ron M. Walls, "Supporting the Health Care Workforce during the COVID-19 Global Epidemic," *JAMA* 323, no. 15 (March 12, 2020), https://jamanetwork .com/journals/jama/fullarticle/2763136.

39. Rabbi Y. Y. Halberstam (Sanzer Rebbe), *"Sikkun oh Tziur Atzmi Avur Chaveiro HaCholeh,"* *BiShvilei HaRefuah* 6, 32–23, and Responsa *Divrei Yatziv*, CM 79(38); and Rabbi D. O. Kleinman, Responsa *Bigdei Chamudot, LiTekufat Choli Korona*, YD 65.

40. To ensure that people would not be discouraged from entering a health care profession out of fear that they would be liable for damages caused while practicing medicine, the Talmud (*Sanhedrin* 74a) rules that if one accidentally damaged property while rushing to save life, they are not required to pay damages. This is also why the rabbis allowed returning home from lifesaving missions on Shabbat and allowed midwives to be paid for their work on Shabbat; see discussion in *Shiurei Torah LeRofim* 2:124, 396–97, 400, and 6:340–41, 133, 137. For this reason, Rabbi Elyashiv ruled that a health care professional woken up to rush to an emergency may take the time necessary to get properly dressed since otherwise no one would want to go into a health care profession. *Shiurei Torah LeRofim* 2:124, 396. Similarly, Rabbi M. Feinstein allows doctors to charge high fees since otherwise people wouldn't dedicate themselves to the study of medicine. *Iggerot Moshe*, YD 4:52. All of this applies to both Jewish and non-Jewish doctors. *Shiurei Torah LeRofim* 6:341, 138.

41. Satmar Rebbe, quoted in *Shiurei Torah LeRofim* 1:10, 130; and anonymous opinion quoted in Responsa *Yaskil Avdi* 6, YD 18(1); *Nishmat Avraham*, YD 336:5 (470 in 3rd ed.) and EH 80:1 (316 in 3rd ed.) in the name of Rabbi Elyashiv (see also *Kovetz Teshuvot* 1:124) and Rabbi Neuvirt. I thank Rabbi M. Torczyner for pointing out this source: Rabbi Mordechai Torczyner, "Charging for Healthcare, Part 1: Accepting Payment, Socialized Medicine," *YUTorah Online*, December 8, 2014, https://www.yutorah.org/sidebar/lecture.cfm/821955/rabbi-morde chai-torczyner/charging-for-healthcare-part-1-accepting-payment-socialized-medicine/; see also extensive discussion of this ruling in Avrohom Blaivas, "May a Doctor Refuse to See Patients," *Journal of Halacha and Contemporary Society*, no. 38 (1999): 100. Rabbi O. Hadaya also rules that a doctor is entitled to breaks since when a patient is not dangerously ill one is not expected to exhaust all their resources or grow weak or injure oneself to treat a patient since the Torah's "ways are ways of pleasantness" and "your life takes precedence." Responsa *Yaskil Avdi* 6, YD18. Rabbi Zilberstein writes that if a doctor is on a break and

someone asks for help, if they can easily and quickly help them, they should, but if it requires a full examination, they are not required to do so. *Shiurei Torah LeRofim* 1, 83.

42. *Shulchan Arukh*, CM 337:19.

43. As argued by Rabbi M. Torczyner "Charging for Healthcare, Part 1."

44. See *Tzitz Eliezer* 5:23, *Minchat Yitzchak* 3:105, and discussion in Noam Salamon, "Concierge Medicine in Halacha," in *And You Shall Surely Heal: The Albert Einstein College of Medicine Synagogue Compendium of Torah and Medicine*, ed. Jonathan Wiesen (New York: The Michael Scharf Publication Trust of the Yeshiva University, 2009), 289–90.

45. See discussion in Prathyusha Chowdri, "What Is Patient Abandonment?" NOLO, n.d., https://www.nolo.com/legal-encyclopedia/what-patient-abandonment.html.

46. See extensive discussions in Mark R. Wicclair, *Conscientious Objection in Health Care: An Ethical Analysis* (Cambridge: Cambridge University Press, 2011), and chapter 7 of this book.

47. *Encyclopedia of Bioethics*, 1:313.

48. William Malouf, "Redefining Professionalism in an Era of Residency Work-Hour Limitations," *AMA Journal of Ethics* 17, no. 2 (2015): 125–26.

49. *Encyclopedia of Bioethics*, 1:314.

50. David Orentlicher, "The Physician's Duty to Treat during Pandemics," *American Journal of Public Health* 108, no. 11 (November 2018): 1459; and Malm et al, "Ethics, Pandemics, and the Duty to Treat," 16.

51. Orentlicher, "Physician's Duty," 16.

52. For example, Rabbi Zilberstein rules that even if a wife doesn't want her husband to leave home to see seriously ill patients, he must do so, even if it is only to reduce the patient's suffering, not to save their life. *Shiurei Torah LeRofim* 1:5, 96–97. See also *Sanhedrin* 73a.

53. Deut. 22:2; *Sifrei Devarim* 22:3; *Bava Kamma* 81b; *Sanhedrin* 73a; and Rambam commentary to Mishnah, *Nedarim* 4:4.

54. See discussion in Freedman, *Duty and Healing*, 149. See also Rabbi Zilberstein, *Shiurei Torah LeRofim* 1:8, 116.

55. Rabbi Elyashiv is quoted as ruling that the verse "You shall give it back" does not require striving for the best possible treatment if the healthcare professional will be harmed as a result. *Shiurei Torah LeRofim* 1:9, 120 and 2:89, 170.

56. Although a medical professional is required to sacrifice their livelihood in order to save a life (*Bava Metzia* 62a), one is not required to sacrifice their livelihood for the sake of a non–dangerously ill patient because the laws of returning a lost object require one to save their own property before that of others (*Bava Metzia* 30b and 33a). Rashi explains that one may go "above and beyond" and sacrifice their own possession in order to return someone else's lost object; see *Shiurei Torah LeRofim* 1:3, 80 and 1:24, 248. Rabbi Zilberstein rules (*Shiurei Torah LeRofim* 1:5, 97) that one is not required to provide medical care for a non-dangerously ill patient if doing so would disrupt the peace of their home since there are exemptions in the laws of returning lost objects based on subjective factors, such as social status and what one would want returned to themselves (*Bava Metzia* 30b). These laws also only obligate one to return to others that which they would want returned to themselves; see discussion in *Shiurei Torah LeRofim* 2:119, 358, 374. See also *Shulchan Arukh*, CM 263:3.

57. *Shulchan Arukh*, CM 263:1. See discussion in Freedman, *Duty and Healing*, 149.

58. *Nedarim* 39b.

59. *Bava Metzia* 30a.

60. *Ahavat Chesed* 3:3n1. See, however, *Chokhmat Shlomo*, CM 426.

61. *Ketubot* 50a.

62. *Minchat Asher* on *Bereishit*, 58 (9), 456.

63. *Minchat Asher* on *Bereishit*, 58 (9), 456.

64. For example, one who does not have an *Etrog* on *Sukkot*, or any other passing mitzvah, is not required to spend more than a fifth of their wealth to acquire one (Rema, OC 656:1). See also *Arukh HaShulchan*, YD 249:5, which says that to give more than one-fifth to do a mitzvah is not pious but forbidden.

65. Responsa *Minchat Asher* 3:42; and Rabbi C. P. Sheinberg, *"BeDin Choleh UMitzta'er Be-Mitzvot,"* *Halakhah URefuah* 4, 135A. See also responsum of Rabbi H. Schachter that one was not required to endanger themselves by performing a ritual cleansing on the dead during the COVID-19 pandemic for this reason.

66. *Iggerot Moshe EH* 3:26(4); *Minchat Asher* on *Bereishit*, 58 (2); and Rabbi M. Feinstein, *Iggerot Moshe* 1:172, as explained by Rabbi O. Yosef in Responsa *Chazon Ovadia* 2:33, 630. For this reason, Rabbi Dovid Cohen rules that if one who has a troubled relationship with their parents that is adversely affecting their emotional health and long-term stability, they may disregard their parents' requests or even disengage entirely from their parents in order to heal since one's emotional health and stability are more valuable than a fifth of their wealth. Yitzchak Schechter, *Kuntres Harofeh LeShevurei Lev: Psychotherapy in Halachah* (New York: printed by the author, 2021), 104–5. See also discussion in Chaim Rappaport, *Judaism and Homosexuality: An Authentic Orthodox View* (London: Vallentine Mitchell, 2004), 93.

67. *Minchat Asher, Bereishit* 58 (8), 453; see also discussions in Lichtenstein, *Headlines 2*, 24–28; and Rabbi Zilberstein, *Shiurei Torah LeRofim*, 2, 372–76, and 6, 353.

68. See extensive discussion in Lichtenstein, *Headlines 2*, 28.

69. See Jason Weiner, "Is There a Right to Healthcare? Towards a Comprehensive Jewish Approach," *Canopy Forum*, July 1, 2020, https://canopyforum.org/2020/07/01/is-there-a-right-to-healthcare-towards-a-comprehensive-jewish-approach/.

70. *Minchat Asher, Bereishit* 58 (8). Rabbi S. Z. Auerbach argues that if someone witnesses another in immediate urgent danger, they should do everything they can to save them, whereas one can contribute toward the communal effort to care for people who are known to be ill but is not required to spend everything they have on their behalf. Responsa *Minchat Shlomo* 2:7(4). Rabbi B. Lau argues, based on *Tosafot, Bava Batra* 10b, that even when there are official frameworks which bear communal responsibility, this does not excuse individuals from protesting injustices in the community. Michael J. Harris, Daniel Rynhold, and Tamra Wright, eds., *Radical Responsibility: Celebrating the Thoughts of Chief Rabbi Lord Jonathan Sacks* (New Milford, CT: Maggid, 2012), 62.

71. Responsa *Minchat Asher* 3:42 (4 and 7). Rabbi Weiss rules that it is forbidden for a person to put their life, or even a limb, in danger to do a mitzvah, and it would not be pious to try to do so, but if doing a mitzvah could cause only non-life-threatening danger, although they are not required, it may be considered pious if they do so anyway. See also

*Minchat Asher, Klalei HaMitzvot*, 15 (5); Rabbi Sheinberg, "*BeDin Choleh UMitzta'er BeMitzvot*," 125, 130, 137–38; and Rabbi Halberstam, "*Sikkun oh Tziur Atzmi Avur Chaveiro HaCholeh*," 6–7, 27, 33.

72. Responsa *Minchat Asher* 3:42; *Minchat Asher, Bereishit*, 59; Rabbi Sheinberg, "*BeDin Choleh UMitzta'er BeMitzvot*," 130, 137–38; Rabbi Y. Y. Halberstam (Sanzer Rebbe), "*Sikkun oh Tziur Atzmi Avur Chaveiro HaCholeh*," 27, 33; and Responsa *Divrei Yatziv*, CM 79.

73. Jason Mills, Jonathan Ramachenderan, Michael Chapman, Rohan Greenland, and Meera Agar, "Prioritizing Workforce Wellbeing and Resilience: What Covid-19 Is Reminding Us about Self-Care and Staff Support," *Palliative Medicine* 34, no. 9 (2020): 1–3.

74. Anne Hofmeyer, Ruth Taylor, and Kate Kennedy, "Fostering Compassion and Reducing Burnout: How Can Health System Leaders Respond in the COVID-19 Pandemic and Beyond?" *Nurse Education Today* 94 (November 2020), https://doi.org/10.1016/j.nedt.2020.104502.

75. Interestingly, one bioethicist has proposed a similar monetary framework for setting realistic limits on the scope of obligations of beneficence by suggesting a round percentage of one's income, such as 10 percent, as a conceptual limit to how far one should be expected to go for others. Peter Singer, *Practical Ethics*, 2nd ed. (Cambridge: Cambridge University Press, 1993), 246.

76. Richard J. Arneson, "Moral Limits on the Demands of Beneficence?" in *The Ethics of Assistance: Morality, Affluence and the Distant Needy*, ed. Deen K. Chatterjee (Cambridge: Cambridge University Press, 2004).

# Conclusion

Developing a world built on the values discussed in this book is a task that cannot be achieved by any one individual or even one generation alone. As our sages remind us, "It is not for you to complete the task, but neither are you free to stand aside from it."[1] While there are limits to how much any individual can accomplish, we are charged with using our own personal gifts and place in the world to contribute as much as we can to our society.[2]

The message of this book is simple but important. How we see the world and our role in it can have a huge impact on the decisions we make and our interactions with others. Approaching life with a desire to give and a sense of responsibility for serving others can transform all of our waking moments into dreams come true. Conversely, when one focuses narrowly on their own rights and taking from others, life can become a nightmare for everyone. A Jewish bioethic of responsibility can be actualized both individually and societally.

Each chapter in this book provides concrete examples of how a compassionate, duty-based approach can be implemented in contemporary health care. Certainly, these same values can be applied to many more areas of life, helping to make the world a better and more just place for all. This goal can be achieved by asking the question "What is my obligation?" whenever challenges arise rather than "What is owed to me?" This change in perspective can have huge ramifications. For us, perhaps the greatest reward is the realization that we are here to give, and in doing so, we live a life of blessing. This is why the influential psychiatrist and Holocaust survivor, Viktor Frankl, recommended that the Statue of Liberty on the East Coast be supplemented by a "Statue of Responsibility" on the West Coast.[3]

An observant Jewish respondent to a qualitative study about COVID-19 vaccines made the claim that "the Torah does not require people to endanger themselves for other peoples' benefit."[4] I hope this book has successfully made the case that such a statement is categorically false.

Rabbi Yekutiel Yehuda Halberstam, scion of the famous Sanz rabbinic dynasty, lost his wife and all eleven of his children in the gas chambers of

Auschwitz. In July of 1944, Rabbi Halberstam was forced to march to the infamous Dachau death camp, during which he and the other frail inmates were made to walk twenty kilometers a day. Those who could not keep up were instantly shot by the SS guards. Indeed, one day Rabbi Halberstam was shot in the shoulder and lost a considerable amount of blood, but seeking medical attention was not an option. As he was losing his strength, he took on himself a vow to God: "If I merit to survive, I will garner all my energies to build a hospital in the Holy Land, where every human being will receive the same dedicated medical care irrespective of nationality or creed." At that moment he noticed a tree with lush green leaves by the side of the road. He reached up, plucked a large leaf, and with his last bit of strength managed to place it on his wound.[5]

The rabbi survived. He never had the opportunity to observe the traditional Jewish mourning rituals for his family because, despite all that he had lost, he felt that the duty to protect and care for those still alive took precedence; thus, he became a leader to the suffering Jews in the displaced persons camps, inspiring them not to give up. After the war he initially went to Brooklyn, New York, where he took it on himself to establish schools, care for orphans, perform weddings, and start a synagogue primarily for other Holocaust survivors in the Beth Moses Hospital.

The prayers in that synagogue were known for being very intense, with no talking whatsoever, and individuals frequently weeping aloud. One Shabbat morning in the summer of 1952, the Torah reader began to chant the weekly portion, which included the section known as the "chastisement" (*tokhechah*),[6] detailing the curses that would befall the Jewish people.[6] It is customary to chant that section very quietly and rapidly, but that morning the rabbi suddenly called out, "*Hekher!*" (louder!). The Torah reader couldn't believe that the rabbi would want him to read that section loudly, so he continued to quickly whisper it in an undertone, but the rabbi demanded, banging on the table, "*Ikh hob gezogt hekher!*" (I said louder!). People began to tremble and cry, so the rabbi explained, "Let the Master of the Universe hear! We have nothing to be afraid of. We have already received all of the curses—and more. Let the Almighty hear, and let Him understand that the time has come to send the blessings!"

Once the prayers had concluded, the rabbi lovingly explained to his congregation that the blessings would come, as God had promised, but that these must result from their own initiatives to be a blessing to the world. He then explained to his congregants that in the coming week, they were to pack their bags one last time and with him to the Land of Israel, where they could help support the fledging community of their fellow survivors in Netanya.

Soon after Rabbi Halberstam and his followers arrived in Netanya and began building a community, the rabbi noticed that this rapidly growing city had no community hospital. It was then that the rabbi took the initiative to uphold the vow he had made during that fateful march a decade earlier. In 1958 the cornerstone was laid for a modern general hospital to serve the entire city, thereby fulfilling the rabbi's pledge to be a blessing. Today that hospital, Laniado, is an important regional medical center.

Rabbi Halberstam was clearly an extraordinary person, but his story—and the ethic of compassionate responsibility developed in this book—can remind us, in the words of Rabbi Jonathan Sacks, that "by making extraordinary demands, [Judaism] inspires ordinary people to live extraordinary lives."[7]

# NOTES

1. *Pirkei Avot* 2:21.

2. For example, Rabbi Soloveitchik argues that creativity creates human responsibility and that a person who "builds hospitals, discovers therapeutic techniques, and saves lives is blessed with dignity" because our limited control over nature enables humanity to achieve dignity and makes it possible to act in accordance with our responsibilities. Joseph B. Soloveitchik, "Lonely Man of Faith," *Tradition* 2, no. 7 (1965): 13.

3. Viktor Frankl, *Man's Search for Meaning*, 4th ed. (Boston: Beacon Press, 1992), 134.

4. Ben Kasstan, "If a Rabbi Did Say 'You Have to Vaccinate,' We Wouldn't: Unveiling the Secular Logics of Religious Exemption and Opposition to Vaccination," *Social Science & Medicine* 280 (July 2021): 4.

5. "A Historical Perspective of Laniado Hospital," American Friends of Laniado Hospital, n.d., http://www.laniadohospital.org/historical-perspective/.

6. The story shared here is as told in Shlomo Riskin, *Listening to God: Inspirations Stories for My Grandchildren* (New Milford, CT: Maggid, 2010), 60.

7. Jonathan Sacks, *To Heal a Fractured World: The Ethics of Responsibility* (New York: Schocken, 2005), 10.

# Index

# About the Author

Rabbi Jason Weiner, DBe, BCC, serves as the senior rabbi and director of the Spiritual Care Department at Cedars-Sinai in Los Angeles. He has earned two rabbinic ordinations as well as a doctorate in clinical bioethics from Loyola University (Chicago), where he also earned a master's degree in bioethics and health policy in addition to a master's degree in Jewish history from Yeshiva University. Rabbi Weiner has completed four units of clinical pastoral education and is a board-certified chaplain. He is a member of the executive committee of the Cedars-Sinai Bioethics Committee. He is past president of the Southern California Board of Rabbis and has been honored with Rabbinic Leadership Awards from the Orthodox Union and Chai Lifeline. He is also the rabbi of Knesset Israel Synagogue of Beverlywood and teaches hands-on Jewish medical ethics in the hospital to numerous Jewish high schools in Los Angeles. He is the author of *Jewish Guide to Practical Medical Decision-Making* (Urim Press) and *Guide to Observance of Jewish Law in a Hospital* (Kodesh Press).